# 32 Days to a
# 32-Inch Waist

## OTHER BOOKS OF INTEREST

### By Ellington Darden, Ph.D.

The Nautilus Diet

The Six-Week Fat-to-Muscle Makeover

High-Intensity Bodybuilding

The Nautilus Book
(REVISED EDITION)

The Nautilus Bodybuilding Book
(REVISED EDITION)

The Athlete's Guide to Sports Medicine

Nutrition for Athletes

Conditioning for Football

Strength-Training Principles

Massive Muscles in 10 Weeks

Big Arms in Six Weeks

100 High-Intensity Ways
to Improve Your Bodybuilding

For a free catalog of
Dr. Darden's fitness books,
please send a
self-addressed, stamped envelope to
Dr. Ellington Darden
Nautilus Sports/Medical Industries
P.O. Box 809014
Dallas, TX 75380-9014.

# 32 Days to a
# 32-Inch Waist

## ELLINGTON DARDEN, PH.D.

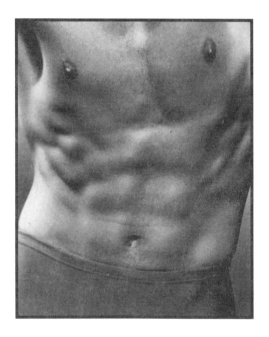

**TAYLOR PUBLISHING COMPANY**
**Dallas, Texas**

Published by
Taylor Publishing Company
1550 West Mockingbird Lane
Dallas, Texas 75235

DESIGNED BY
LURELLE CHEVERIE

COMPOSITION BY
HIGH RESOLUTION, INC.

Library of Congress
Cataloging-in-Publication Data

Darden, Ellington, 1943-
      32 days to a 32-inch waist / by Ellington Darden.
         p.   cm.
      ISBN 0–87833–710–5 : $8.95
         1. Low-calorie diet.   2. Reducing exercises.   3. Exercise for men.
   I. Title.   II. Title: Thirtytwo days to a thirtytwo-inch waist.
   RM222.2.D289   1990                              89-71364
   613.2'5—dc20                                         CIP

Printed in the United States of America

10   9   8   7   6   5   4

## ACKNOWLEDGMENTS

Many people deserve thanks for their
contributions to this book.

**Connie May**   did an excellent job of editing the text.

**Brenda Hutchins**   planned the menus and shopping lists.

**Ken Hutchins**   took many of the before-and-after
photographs, and assisted with much of
the research on super-slow exercise.

**Dan Howard**   took the front cover photograph as
well as the exercise pictures.

**Blake Boyd**   demonstrated the recommended
exercises and volunteered his lean waist
for the front cover.

**Bob Sikora, Connie May, Jerry Coronado, Brenda Smedley,
Claude Howell, Mark Spradling,** and **Diane Travis**
trained the men involved in the
32/32 research in Dallas.

My sincere appreciation goes to those
mentioned above, and to all the men who participated
in the research for this project.

# CONTENTS

# =1=
# So . . . You Want a 32-Inch Waist

A 32-inch waistline!

Sounds great, doesn't it?

When you graduated from high school, you probably had a smaller waist, a flatter stomach, and no "love handles" on your sides.

Your former physique doesn't have to be a thing of the past. By properly applying the information in this book, you can make your midsection as trim and firm as it was in high school—in a little more than a month!

In some cultures, big-bellied men are admired. That's not often the case in the United States. There is no great demand in this country for the John Candy look. A big gut today makes climbing the corporate ladder more difficult. A lean waist—besides the obvious health benefits—denotes discipline, motivation, and patience.

Obtaining that ever-elusive 32-inch waist requires what most men hate: *diet and exercise.*

But what type of diet and exercise? With over 29,000 choices available, the typical overfat person could try a different plan for the next seventy-nine years and not come close to exhausting his options.

For over twenty years, I have been researching a diet and exercise program that has shown impressive results. The program combines a descending-calorie diet with high-intensity exercise. The scientific blending of these factors in 32/32 permits you to lose fat and build muscle at the same time, so that you look better in a shorter period of time.

Simultaneously losing fat and building muscle creates an important synergistic effect that produces guaranteed fat loss, increased metabolic rate, and improved body shape. I'll thoroughly discuss these factors in Chapter 8, but let me emphasize that losing fat and building muscle *at the same time* is the key to achieving and maintaining a 32-inch waist.

You'll be guided through this program by easy-to-follow, scientifically-designed menus, recipes, exercises, and helpful hints that have worked for thousands of men. In 1988, I worked with 146 men in Dallas, Texas, who were carefully supervised through the exact eating and exercise plan you'll be following.

Let's review what several of the men experienced during the 32/32 program.

## GOOD-BYE SOFT AND BLOATED FEELING

Mark Spradling is a 29-year-old computer systems administrator in Dallas. He entered the program weighing 157 pounds at a height of 5 feet 9 inches. His body-fat level was 15 percent and his waist measured 32⅝ inches. With a slightly smaller than average build, he looked okay.

"But even though I was in fairly good condition when I started the course," remembers Mark, "I still felt soft and bloated around the midsection. I needed some specific guidance on what to eat and how to exercise."

The 32/32 program met Mark's needs perfectly. He lost 23 pounds of fat and built 3 pounds of muscle. His waist measurement dropped 4 inches to an incredibly small 28⅝ inches, which better fit his frame.

"Being single," Mark notes, "my cooking and eating habits were always haphazard. The 32/32 meals taught me about calories and their importance in reshaping the body. I now know how to shop purposefully, make wise selections of food, and prepare them in a healthy way.

"Plus, I've become addicted to the benefits of intense exercise. I'm eager to put on more muscle."

Putting on more muscle is exactly what Mark did in subsequent months. Keeping his body fat at a low percentage, Mark was able to add another 7 pounds of muscle to his lean physique.

**"I never thought my waist would be this small again."**

## MARK SPRADLING
### age 29

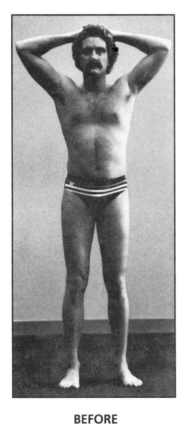

Lost
23
pounds
of fat

Built
3
pounds
of muscle

AND
TRIMMED
4
inches off
his waist

in
32 days!

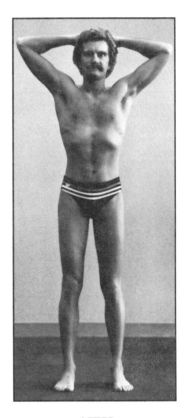

| **BEFORE** | **AFTER** |
|:---:|:---:|
| Waist Size: | Waist Size: |
| 32⁵/₈ | 28⁵/₈ |

"People used to joke about my 'pregnancy.' After a while, I realized that the only thing I was expecting was heart problems, shortness of breath, a sore back, and low self-esteem. I decided it was time to give birth to a new body. Now people are envious, and that's no joke!"

### KEN HOWELL
### age 59

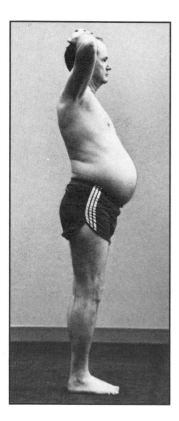

Lost
36¼
pounds
of fat

Built
7¾
pounds
of muscle

AND
TRIMMED
10¾
inches off
his waist

in
96 days!

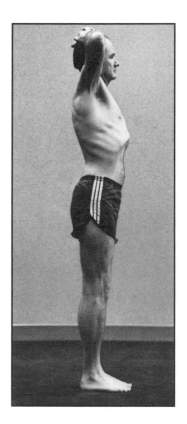

**BEFORE**
Waist Size:
42½

**AFTER**
Waist Size:
31¾

## NO MORE POT BELLY

Of the 146 men who have been through the 32/32 program in Dallas, no one made more spectacular changes in his body than 59-year-old Ken Howell. An engineer at Texas Instruments, Ken went through the program three times, losing 36¼ pounds of fat and gaining 7¾ pounds of muscle. His waist measurement shrank from 42½ to 31¾—a reduction of 10¾ inches.

"I feel like a new man," Ken smiles. "In fact, I rolled over in bed last night, and for the first time in over ten years I realized my pot belly was gone. I could actually lie on my stomach without getting seasick from balancing on my belly."

Ken was encouraged to join the program by his wife, Claude, who had been through a similar program for women. "I was so elated with my results that I just had to get Kenneth involved," recalls Claude.

"All my clothes are being altered," says Ken. "But it's worth the cost. With my new body I feel a hundred percent stronger and much more energetic."

Although Ken did not achieve a 32-inch waist in 32 days, he had the patience to continue with the program. After 96 days, he exceeded his goal.

## REMOVING THOSE
## LOVE HANDLES

Jim Graham wanted to get rid of his love handles. A 31-year-old real estate broker and avid golfer, Jim started the program with a 35-inch waist. At a height of 6 feet, his body weight was 190 pounds.

After 32 days of dieting and thirteen high-intensity exercise sessions, Jim lost 22 pounds of fat and gained 3½ pounds of muscle. From his waistline alone he lost 4⅛ inches.

"I thought I'd just have to learn to live with my love handles," Jim laughed as he unsuccessfully tried to pull an inch of flesh from his side. "Now, I realize all it takes is proper diet and proper exercise."

"My clothes fit much better now that I've lost my excess fat. My friends have made favorable comments on my healthy appearance, my wife is very pleased, and my golf game has improved. What more could I ask?"

Jim's waistline is now smaller than when he was in high school.

*"*The program taught me how to select foods wisely and prepare them in a nutritious, low-calorie manner.*"*

## JIM GRAHAM
### age 31

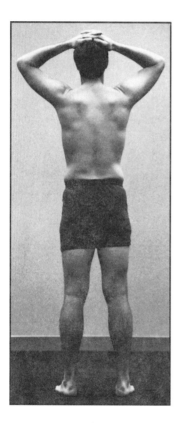

Lost
22
pounds
of fat

Built
3½
pounds
of muscle

AND
TRIMMED
4⅛
inches off
his waist

in
32 days!

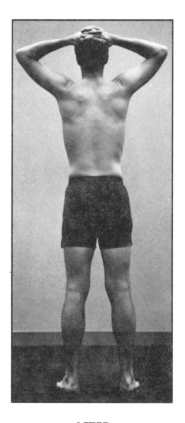

**BEFORE**
Waist Size:
35

**AFTER**
Waist Size:
30⅞

## GET SERIOUS

Mark, Ken, and Jim admit that slimming and muscularizing the waist through diet and exercise takes work. But like most other meaningful accomplishments in life, the results are worth the effort.

This book offers no magic formulas, no easy solutions, no painless pills. Instead, it provides you with a well-balanced, lower-calorie eating plan combined with high-intensity exercise routines. Gradually, your fat will be removed, your muscles strengthened, and your health improved. The process takes discipline and patience, and the principles in this book.

It's time to think—and act—seriously about a 32-inch waist!

# =2=

# Spot Reduction—
# What Really Matters

Before going deeper into this book, I'd like to clear up a lingering misconception about bellyfat and love handles: *spot reduction*.

Spot reduction is the idea that when you exercise a specific body part, such as the abdominals, the involved muscles use the surrounding fat for energy. This belief is the reason high-repetition sit-ups, side bends, leg raises, and twisting movements have been practiced for years as a way to remove fat from the waist. Unfortunately, such beliefs and practices are not based on scientific fact.

## THE FACTS ABOUT SPOT REDUCTION

The fat that is stored around your waist is in a form called lipids. To be used as energy, the lipids must first be converted to fatty acids. This is a very complex chemical procedure. To be used as fuel, the lipids travel through the bloodstream to the liver. In the liver they are converted to fatty acids, which are then transported to the working muscles.

This would be convenient if the fat cells selected were from areas where you have the thickest layers. But a problem arises because no direct pathways exist from the fat cells to the muscle cells. When fat is used for energy, it is mobilized primarily through the liver from multiple fat cells all over the body. The selection process your body uses for mobilizing its fat stores is genetically programmed. The mobilization process, in fact, is in the reverse order from which you store fat. The last places you usually store fat are the first from which you lose it.

A typical man, for example, deposits fat first on the sides of his waist. It usually goes over the navel area second, then the hips, the back, and

**8**

finally the thighs. When he starts losing fat, it comes off in reverse order—thighs, back, hips, navel area, and finally his sides.

Each person has a slightly different ordering of fat-storage spots. But that ordering is genetically determined and not subject to change.

Spot reduction, therefore, is physiologically impossible. Those performing or recommending specific spot-reducing exercises are misinformed.

## SUPPORTIVE RESEARCH

Several scientific studies support the fact that spot reduction is *not* possible. One such study measured the skinfold thicknesses of the arms of accomplished tennis players. If spot reduction were feasible, the more active—or playing—arms of the players would be significantly leaner than their inactive arms. Both arms of these tennis players were shown to be equal in fat content.

An even more convincing study compared the effect of abdominal training on fat-cell size. Abdominal, gluteal, and subscapular fat biopsies were taken from fifteen experimental and six control subjects before and after a 27-day abdominal exercise program.

Some subjects performed as many as five thousand sit-ups during this program. The results showed that fat cell diameters decreased significantly at all three sampling sites, but there were no significant differences in the rate of change among the various areas. This research supports the fact that specific exercises, such as sit-ups, do not preferentially reduce abdominal fat cell size.

## WHAT MATTERS MOST

What really matters in losing fat efficiently are four concepts:

1. The overall consumption of dietary calories must be lower than the energy expenditure on a daily basis.

2. The dietary calories should be well balanced from the major food groups.

3. The dietary calories should descend gradually as the diet progresses.

4. Combined with the three dietary facts above is the importance of muscle-building exercise to assure guaranteed fat loss, increased metabolic rate, and improved body shape.

Even with the application of the above facts, it is important to understand that fat losses come from throughout the body in disproportionate amounts according to individual genetics.

## SPOT REDUCTION, NO—
## SPOT PRODUCTION, YES!

While it is not possible for you to spot reduce fat cells around your waist, it is possible to spot produce muscular size and strength in selective body parts.

Isolating and strengthening the right muscles can reduce flabbiness on your waist, give greater definition to your thighs and hips, broaden your shoulders, deepen your chest, muscularize your upper arms, and add overall confidence to your walk.

In other words, to get your waistline down to 32 inches requires intense exercise for most of your major muscles combined with a well-balanced, descending-calorie diet.

That's exactly what is in store for you over the next 32 days.

# _=3=_
# Just 32 Days

There are several reasons why 32 days works well in this diet and exercise program.

*First*, 32 days is only one or two days longer than a month, which is a reasonable time period for people to diet.

*Second*, 32 days divides evenly into four 8-day segments, or two 16-day periods. This allows for an effective way to repeat and rotate the menus.

*Third*, in 32 days you can exercise thirteen times and still have an average of two-and-one-half day's rest between each workout. Such a schedule seems to promote maximum muscular growth stimulation in untrained men.

*Fourth*, 32/32 not only gets a man's attention, but it's an acronym for the book's central idea: 32 Days to a 32-Inch Waist.

The 32/32 program you're about to embark on may be demanding at times, but you won't be traveling alone. Hundreds of men thriving on hard work and achievement have been there before you. And hundreds more will follow.

You will meet the challenges—and reach your goals—if you follow the menus and exercises in the subsequent chapters.

# _=4=_

# Great Expectations: Losses and Gains

How much can you expect to lose if you follow the program diligently for 32 days? Examining the average losses of the men involved in my research should provide insight.

## 32/32 RESEARCH

The 32/32 program was last tested with 146 men in Dallas, Texas. The average participant was 39.57 years old, 69.85 inches tall, and had a starting body weight of 198.44 pounds. Their overall results were impressive.

Each man lost an average of:

- 17.07 pounds of fat

- 3.03 inches off the waist

- 1.73 inches off the hips

- 2.65 inches off the thighs

The men simultaneously added an average of 3.65 pounds of muscle to their bodies. These numbers provide realistic expectations for men motivated to follow the 32-day course of action.

## REACHING THE GOAL

The men who regained 32-inch waists were thrilled to fit into clothes they had previously outgrown. A few complained, albeit proudly, about the costs of alterations. Others looked forward to purchasing new wardrobes.

Most men whose goals were beyond those obtainable in 32 days vowed to continue with the program, either on their own or by formally reentering. A few realized they would never achieve a 32-inch waist because of their bone structure, but each was encouraged by his fat loss and muscle gain.

## REALISTIC PROJECTIONS

If you're an average man weighing approximately 200 pounds, at a height of 5 feet 10 inches, you can expect to lose from 15 to 20 pounds of fat, reduce 3 inches from your waist, and add 3$\frac{1}{2}$ pounds of muscle overall. A 32-inch waist for you in 32 days is an achievable goal.

If you weigh significantly more or less than 200 pounds, however, your overall results may vary considerably. The principles involved in this course still apply, but it may take you more or fewer days to reach your goal.

Keep your projections realistic. Act now. And profit with fat losses!

# =5=

# Your Waist from the Inside Out

Fat stomach, flat stomach, big stomach, small stomach.

You often hear the word *stomach* used in the context above. Actually, stomach is a term more accurately describing your digestive organ. Descriptive terms for the area of the body men worry so much about are *waist* and *midsection*.

Anatomically speaking, your waist or midsection is the area between your breastbone and pelvis. Let's take a close look at what composes your waist, from the inside out.

## INTERNAL ORGANS

In the upper middle of your waist, tucked under your diaphragm, are your stomach and liver. Slightly underneath these two organs lies your pancreas. Below your stomach is the small intestine, which twists around in the center of your midsection at approximately the level of your navel and finally connects to the large intestine or colon.

Intermingled are millions of fat cells, each capable of becoming a storage depot for excess calories.

## FOUR IMPORTANT MIDSECTION MUSCLES

Sheathing your internal cells and organs are four layers of muscle that have several important functions. They support and protect your organs, and they help to keep your pelvis in proper alignment.

Each of the four midsection muscles permits a different movement. The fibers of the innermost muscle, the *transverse abdominis*, stretch across the waist from side to side. When the transverse muscles contract they compress the internal organs, assisting in breathing out and with the normal process of elimination.

On top of the transverse abdominis is the *internal oblique*. These muscle fibers start at the hip and run diagonally upward to meet the lower ribs. Lateral flexion and torso rotation to the same side are the main functions of the internal oblique muscles.

The next layer is the *external oblique*, a wide but thin muscle originating at the borders of the lower ribs and extending forward and downward. These fibers run at right angles to those of the inner muscle. The primary function of the external oblique is to bend the spine to the same side and to rotate the torso to the opposite side.

The outermost layer of muscle, the *rectus abdominis*, stretches vertically from the rib cage to the pelvic bone. The function of the rectus abdominis is to shorten the distance between the breastbone and the pelvic girdle. To feel this muscle, lie flat on your back with your knees bent and feet flat on the floor. Roll your head and shoulders forward. In this position, if you jab your fingertips into your waist, you can feel the contracted rectus abdominis underneath the skin.

Between the skin and the superficial muscles—the rectus in front and the external oblique on the sides—are layers of fat, the thickness of which depends on your genetics and percent of body fat.

## LOWER BACK MUSCLES

The back of your waist holds your spine and several large muscles, primarily the *psoas major, quadratus lumborium, erector spinae,* and *latissimus dors*i. When the muscles of your lower back and the muscles of your waist are strong, they work together to create a tight supportive girdle around the spine.

Weak midsection muscles encourage the spine to sag toward the front of the body, which may lead to injury. Strong waist muscles help you to maintain a healthy, upright posture, and to perform better in sports and recreational activities.

## PROPER DIET
## AND PROPER EXERCISE

Now that you have some understanding of what's behind your navel, you can see why your major muscles respond rapidly to exercise. But it takes more than a marathon of sit-ups to flatter your midsection. A trim waist requires a scientific approach of proper diet and proper exercise.

# =6=
# Proper Diet

The 32/32 program is successful because it scientifically combines proper diet and proper exercise. The next chapter discusses proper exercise. This chapter details the composition of a proper diet.

## SEVEN CRITERIA

A reducing diet must meet seven criteria. In question form, they are:

- Does the diet provide a reasonable number of calories—an absolute minimum of 1,000 calories a day?

- Does it supply enough but not too much protein—at least the recommended intake of 0.4 grams per pound of body weight, but not more than twice this much?

- Does it provide enough fat for satiety, but not too much, so that between 20 and 35 percent of the day's total calories come from fat?

- Does it supply enough carbohydrate to spare protein, so you won't utilize muscle tissue for energy—about 100 grams of carbohydrate for the average-sized person?

- Does it present a balance of vitamins and minerals from whole food sources in all the Basic Four food groups?

- Does it offer enough variety so that you won't give up on the diet from boredom?

- Does it consist of ordinary foods available in supermarkets at reasonable prices?

**17**

The 32/32 diet plan meets and exceeds all seven criteria. It is not only sound, safe, and effective, but easy to follow and particularly well suited to an intense exercise program.

## SPECIFIC GUIDELINES

Chapters 13 through 16 provide you with specific menus and recipes for each day's meals, together with a shopping list of everything you'll need for each 16-day period.

If you do a lot of outside entertaining, it is possible to adapt the 32/32 plan to restaurant dining. You'll find that the daily menus protect you from between-meal hunger at home or away. The sense of satiety they provide will minimize your temptation to cheat and maximize your fat loss.

Most men use the 32/32 diet as the basis for a new way of eating. They discover their fat-friendly eating patterns are soon replaced by waist-conscious food selections. After you've lost the weight you want to lose, you won't have to stay within the 32/32 calorie limits, but you will find that you can stay happily and healthily with its eating principles for the rest of your life. The 32/32 maintenance plan shows you how to adapt the menus to lifetime eating.

At the heart of the program is a descending-calorie diet. You begin with 1,500 calories a day for 16 days. Then, for days 17 through 32 the calories are reduced to 1,400 per day. As the intensity of the exercise increases, the dietary calories decrease, thus allowing you to build muscle and lose fat simultaneously without feeling worn out. It is the descending-calorie feature that makes this diet particularly good to use in conjunction with the high-intensity routines.

## BASIC FOUR

Another health feature of the 32/32 diet is that it is well balanced. Each day your food is divided into proper proportions of the Basic Four food groups:

- **Meat Group:** meat, poultry, fish, eggs, and legumes such as dried beans, peas, lentils

- **Milk Group:** milk, yogurt, cheese

- **Fruits and Vegetables Group**

- **Breads and Cereals Group:** grains, cereals, rice, pasta

For 32 days, you are given menus designed to meet an approximate 2:2:4:4 ratio of Meat to Milk to Fruits and Vegetables to Breads and Cereals. A 2:2:4:4 ratio means that your daily caloric intake will be approximately 50 percent carbohydrates, 30 percent fats, and 20 percent proteins —a diet pattern good for life. Whether you are dieting or not, the basic proportioning of food groups in the 32/32 plan is the key to eating nutritionally balanced meals.

The emphasis in the Basic Four is on what you should eat. Nutritionists now recognize a fifth food group—labeled "Other"—made up of foods to consume in small amounts. The Other category contains fats, sugars, and alcohol. Consuming these foods may provide you with ample calories but insufficient amounts of essential vitamins and minerals.

Fats, sugars, and alcohol are calorie-dense, providing more calories than nutrients. Fats (such as butter, margarine, oils, and salad dressings) are often referred to as concentrated calories because, gram for gram, they contain more than twice the calories of either proteins or carbohydrates. You should not cut fats from your diet altogether. Moderate amounts of fat provide a feeling of satisfaction, or satiety, which is very important over the long haul because it keeps you on the diet. Part of your fat allotment each day is built into foods from the Basic Four food groups. Milk, meat, and most breads contain fat. In examining the menus, notice that you'll be adding only small quantities of fat to that which you'll be getting from the Basic Four.

## TO GORGE OR GRAZE?

Research shows that nibblers are better off nutritionally than gorgers. Those eating many small meals a day are more efficient at keeping lean. The 32/32 diet has been designed with this principle in mind.

The menus presented in later chapters are composed of the usual meals: breakfast, lunch, and dinner. In addition, there are between-meal snacks to be considered part of your daily food intake. You may choose when to consume the snacks—morning, afternoon, or after dinner—whenever you want the distraction or the comfort of a nibble. Should you want to snack more frequently, subtract foods from lunch and dinner menus to eat between meals.

Think of water as a snack, too. Drink at least twelve glasses of tap, seltzer, or mineral water each day. One of the body's most important nutrients, water can be particularly helpful for dieters because the satiety it provides diminishes feelings of hunger.

Most of the participants I work with in Dallas purchase plastic water bottles, the kind with a straw, readily available in supermarkets, service stations, and convenience stores. With these bottles you can carry water throughout the day for constant drinking. Most trainees find the containers are also perfect for use during exercise sessions.

Limited snacking or nibbling will keep your body's fat-burning mechanism in smooth operation throughout the day.

Eat lightly, and eat often.

# =7=
# Proper Exercise

Many people perceive exercise as "anything involving movement." To them, exercise is playing with the kids, raking the yard, even walking the dog.

Exercise to reshape and maintain your body requires a logical plan to fatigue your major muscles. A proper exercise program involves quantity movement of the body against quality resistance. Muscular fatigue should occur briefly, within one to two minutes. Such exercise mandates consistent recording of movement and resistance progression as performance improves. For these reasons, proper exercise demands training with barbells, dumbbells, or machines such as Nautilus.

## IMPORTANCE OF INTENSITY

The problem with many reducing programs is that the recommended exercise is too low in intensity to effectively stimulate the muscles. Jogging, cycling, swimming, and walking are all ways to improve your cardiovascular fitness and burn calories. But they do not efficiently challenge your muscles to grow larger and stronger. The best way to accomplish this growth is with high-intensity exercise.

A typical high-intensity workout—the kind you'll be performing during the 32/32—lasts for only 20 minutes. But during those 20 minutes you must be willing to give each exercise your ultimate effort. You must make your workout hard, brief, and challenging if you want maximum results.

## ADVANTAGES OF MOVING SLOW

Another important factor in getting maximum results is the speed with which you lift and lower the weights on each repetition. Since 1982, Ken and Brenda Hutchins and I have been researching the effects of performing repetitions in a very slow and deliberate manner. This style of training, "super slow," requires lifting the weight in 10 seconds and lowering it in 5 seconds.

There are three primary advantages of super-slow compared to faster styles of training.

1. **Super slow provides more thorough muscle-fiber involvement**. When you move slowly during a repetition, you significantly reduce the momentum that normally occurs. As a result, you activate parts of the muscle not usually brought into play.

2. **Super slow is safer**. Since you are lifting the weight in a smooth, controlled fashion, there are no sudden starts and stops. The force on the muscle remains steady, providing more structural safety than traditionally fast, jerky styles of lifting.

3. **Super slow produces better strength-building results**. Compared to the traditional way of performing a repetition, super-slow training produces 59 percent better strength gains.

Super-slow training is much more productive at increasing muscular size and strength. As such, it's the ideal complement to a descending-calorie diet.

Naturally, super slow works best when it's performed according to a tried-and-tested protocol.

To explore super slow, try the following on a standard leg extension machine.

## SUPER-SLOW LEG EXTENSIONS

- Sit in the machine, ankles behind the roller pads. Your knees should be bent.

- Try to barely move the resistance, by only a perceptible 1/8 inch.

- Proceed slowly and smoothly once you start moving.

- Continue to straighten your legs at a constant speed to arrive at the fully extended position at the 10-second mark. Initially, someone with a stopwatch should help you with the training.

- Pause momentarily in the extended position.

- Ease out of the top position *gradually*. Smoothly increase your speed on the descent, still moving slowly. It should take you approximately 5 seconds to return to the starting position.

- Let the weight stack touch, but do not rest or let the slack out of the chain. When you feel the weight touch, begin to barely move again in the upward direction.

- Concentrate on keeping the movement arm traveling at a near-constant speed. Do not try to stop and heave into the resistance.

- Keep the lifting slow, but steady. Keep the lowering smooth.

- Stop once you've experienced four or five correct repetitions.

Even in lifting a light weight you should begin to feel a burning sensation in your frontal thighs. Do not be alarmed. The burning is an indication that the involved muscle fibers are being thoroughly activated.

Once you get the rhythm of super slow, select a resistance that permits you to perform between four and eight repetitions. This is the weight you should use for your next session. When you can do eight or more repetitions in good form, increase the resistance at your following workout by approximately 5 percent.

## SUPERIOR RESULTS
## FROM SUPER SLOW

Super slow can be applied to almost any type of weight-training equipment: Nautilus, barbells, dumbbells, or even body weight resistance. The following guidelines apply regardless of which equipment you use.

1. Select three to five exercises for your lower body and five to seven exercises for your upper body—no more than ten exercises in any workout.

2. Exercise not more than three nonconsecutive days per week. High-intensity training necessitates a recovery period of at least 48 hours. Your body gets stronger during rest, not during exercise.

3. Select a resistance for each exercise that allows the performance of four to eight super-slow repetitions.

   a. Start with a weight that you can comfortably lift for four repetitions.

   b. Continue with that weight until eight or more strict repetitions are performed. In your subsequent workout, increase the resistance by 5 percent.

   c. Attempt to increase the number of repetitions or the amount of weight, or both, at each workout. But *do not sacrifice form* in an attempt to produce repetition and resistance improvements.

4. Concentrate during each repetition on lifting the weight slowly in 10 seconds, and lowering it smoothly in 5 seconds.

5. Lift more slowly, not more quickly, if you are in doubt about the speed of movement.

6. Relax body parts that are not involved in each exercise. Pay particular attention to relaxing your face, neck, and.hand muscles.

7. Breathe normally. Try not to hold your breath during any stage of the repetition.

8. Keep accurate written records—date, resistance, repetitions, and overall training time—of each workout.

## THE NAUTILUS ADVANTAGE

If you have access to Nautilus equipment, use it. It's safer and easier to use than barbells and dumbbells. A beginner can learn to use Nautilus equipment correctly and effectively in two or three sessions.

Availability is usually not a problem, as there are more than five thousand specialized Nautilus facilities in the United States. Organizations such as YMCAs, universities and colleges, recreation centers, government agencies, and the Armed Forces may also provide access to Nautilus.

You can, however, complete the 32/32 program without access to Nautilus, employing other brands of weight machines or free weights to duplicate the standard Nautilus exercises. Chapter 19 illustrates a productive workout with free weights.

# =8=
# Synergism

Synergism is the simultaneous occurrence of separate factors that together have greater total effect than the sum of their individual actions. The effects of the 32/32 reducing plan combined with the 32/32 exercises are an excellent example of synergism. Simultaneously losing fat and building muscle produces at least three important results: guaranteed fat loss, increased metabolic rate, and improved body shape.

## GUARANTEED FAT LOSS

Guaranteed fat loss means that weight loss from the diet and exercise program is entirely from fat stores. Most other plans produce weight losses not solely from fat but from significant reductions in fluids and tissues. Losing fluids from muscles, blood, and organs is dangerous. The guaranteed way, and the best way, to ensure that weight loss is completely from fat stores is to stimulate your muscles to grow, using fat as a source of energy.

But how does muscle strengthening guarantee your weight loss will be from fat?

A study published by Dr. Alfred Goldberg and colleagues in a 1975 issue of *Medicine and Science in Sports* details the process. In working with animals, Dr. Goldberg found that if muscle is stimulated to grow through exercise, it will grow in defiance of tremendous adversity—even at the expense of the remainder of the organism.

A fundamental trait of animal life is locomotion, which depends on muscular size and strength. Survival resources are allocated to the muscles first. This priority allocation depends, however, on muscle stimulation. Without that stimulation, resources are stored, passed out, or put to other uses.

In my opinion, the same physiology is in operation within the human body. When you embark on a low-calorie diet, your body perceives that something is wrong. It starts preserving fat as a survival mechanism. To prevent this from occurring, you must overrule your survival mechanism by stimulating muscle growth. Your muscles will then pull calories from your fat cells and your weight loss will be entirely from fat.

## INCREASED METABOLIC RATE

Both muscle and fat require calories for vital functioning. Muscle is very active metabolically. Fat is just the opposite—almost dormant. A gain of one pound of muscle raises your metabolic rate by approximately 75 calories per day. Muscle burns 37.5 times more calories per day than an equal amount of fat, which burns only 2 calories a day per pound.

As your muscles grow larger—as they will from the 32/32 exercise—your metabolic rate will increase. Your new body, with extra muscle and less fat, will burn more calories.

Especially inviting is the fact that your maintenance plan for permanent weight control can include many of your favorite foods and drinks. With additional muscles demanding extra calories daily just for maintenance, you can eat normally without regaining your lost fat.

## IMPROVED BODY SHAPE

Probably the most gratifying result of this program is improved body shape. Body shape is dependent on your muscle-to-fat ratio, and most men over thirty have too little muscle and too much fat. Gaining muscle and losing fat dramatically improves the appearance of your physique—especially your waist. The confidence you have in your physique impacts you physically, mentally, and socially. When you reshape your body through 32/32, you'll look better, feel better, and perform better.

The 32/32 course was designed primarily to give participants the advantages of muscular fitness and the positive mental attitude that can accompany it.

## SYNERGISM IN ACTION

You should now see that the proper application of the 32/32 program will allow you to enhance your own metabolic synergism. You can ascertain that your weight loss is entirely from fat. You can be sure that your muscles are significantly larger and stronger, which will speed up your metabolic rate. And you can revel in the self-confidence your new body shape provides.

# =9=
# Weight-Training Myths

Old myths are hard to dispel. In spite of all the recent news about weight training—its popularity is on the rise, and legitimate research is finally proving many of the benefits of stronger, larger muscles—a great deal of blatant misinformation has survived. Many of the myths are relatively harmless, except that people who believe them deny themselves the strength, leanness, and vitality weight training *could* provide. Following are some common myths you should understand.

## MYTH:
## WEIGHT TRAINING WILL
## MAKE YOU MUSCLE-BOUND.

A stereotype equates muscular development with being stiff, tight, and muscle-bound. It is true that some men with large muscles lack a normal degree of flexibility. Large muscles can be developed through training regimens that do little, if anything, to improve flexibility. In rare cases, the activity that made the muscles larger concurrently produced a loss of flexibility. But in the vast majority of cases, muscle size has a positive correlation to flexibility. When weight training is conducted properly, and especially when Nautilus machines are used, the full-range exercises that improve muscular size and strength simultaneously increase flexibility.

# MYTH:
# WEIGHT TRAINING WILL
# SLOW YOU DOWN.

Just the opposite is true. If everything else is equal, the stronger, larger-muscled person will move faster because he will have a greater muscle mass to body weight ratio. Add more horsepower to the engine of an automobile and it will travel faster even though it weighs more.

Suppose you want to curl a 100-pound barbell as fast as possible. If your biceps muscle is capable of curling exactly 101 pounds, then your speed of movement with 100 pounds will be very slow. Perhaps five seconds will be needed to move from the extended to the flexed position. On the other hand, if your biceps is capable of curling 120 pounds, you'll curl the 100-pound barbell in half a second or less. If your curling capacity is 130 pounds, your speed of movement will be even more rapid. Since skill is not significantly involved in curling a barbell, increases in speed must be accomplished by strengthening the involved muscles.

The same holds true with movements not related to strength training. Any type of muscle-powered movement is met by some kind of resistance: air, water, gravity, or friction. Given equal resistance, the stronger person will invariably be faster.

# MYTH:
# WEIGHT TRAINING DOES
# NOTHING FOR YOUR
# CARDIOVASCULAR SYSTEM.

Under the right circumstances, you can build a high level of cardiovascular endurance from weight training. The conditions required to do so follow.

1. Be sufficiently skilled to perform the exercises, or use the exercise machines, in good form.

2. Have enough strength to elevate your heart rate to 70 to 85 percent of your maximum.

3. Have your equipment arranged so that you can move quickly, in 15 seconds or less, between the end of one exercise and the beginning of the next.

4. Be willing to withstand the discomfort and pain resulting

from having an elevated heart rate, labored breathing, and momentary muscular fatigue all at the same time.

I've trained hundreds of people who were able to achieve high levels of cardiovascular endurance with weight training. I've also experienced it myself. Yet many fitness-minded people still believe that obtaining a high level of cardiovascular endurance from weight training is impossible. Granted, in many facilities crowded conditions prevent you from moving quickly from one machine to the next. When such factors keep you from meeting the above requirements, it may be appropriate to combine weight training with some type of aerobic exercise. But if you can get both muscular and cardiovascular stimulation from one activity, you're much better off.

Furthermore, four major studies have shown that proper weight training produces high levels of cardiovascular endurance. The study by Stephen Messier and Mary Dill in the December 1985 issue of the *Research Quarterly for Exercise and Sport* is particularly informative.

## MYTH: WEIGHT TRAINING TAKES TOO MUCH TIME.

Contrary to popular belief, properly performed weight training takes only 20 minutes per workout. Performed three times per week, that's one hour of training time for every seven days. Investing one hour per week exercising yields the best returns attainable in such a small amount of time.

## MYTH: WEIGHT TRAINING RETARDS FAT LOSS.

Weight training is a valuable adjunct to a reducing diet. Weight training will not only protect your muscle mass but also increase it during your weight-loss period. Dieters who do not exercise with weights invariably lose muscle along with fat, occasionally to the point of losing some heart tissue. It is important to realize that for every pound of muscle lost, your resting metabolic rate decreases by an average of 75 calories per day. Many dieters therefore end up with lower metabolisms. When they return to normal eating patterns, back come the original pounds—and often more.

Strengthening your muscles through weight training speeds up your metabolism so that you can eat reasonably after reducing and stay lean.

# MYTH:
# IF YOU WANT A GOOD WAISTLINE, DO HUNDREDS OF SIT-UPS EACH DAY.

Despite the popular misconception that you can spot reduce a fatty area with lots of targeted exercise, doing high-repetition sit-ups won't make a dent in your midsection. In fact, sit-ups are not highly rated as an exercise for your abdominals. Sit-ups primarily work your *iliopsoas* muscles, or hip flexors. A better exercise for your midsection is the trunk curl, described and illustrated in Chapter 19. To substantially improve your abdominals, you'll also need a lower-calorie diet and the understanding that *fat comes off gradually* from all over your body, not just a few selected spots.

# MYTH:
# RUNNING IS THE BEST OVERALL EXERCISE FOR YOUR WAIST.

Running, done properly, provides excellent cardiovascular endurance but does little for the rest of your body. In running, your legs are involved mostly in their midrange of movement, so their flexibility is not greatly increased. And consider the pounding on your feet and legs. When your feet hit the ground, the ground hits back with a force of three to five times your body weight. Most of this force is transferred to your feet, ankles, and sensitive knee joints. It's easy to understand why most runners have multiple problems with these areas.

The best overall conditioner for your waist is not running, but weight training combined with sensible eating.

## MYTH:
## WEIGHT TRAINING
## INCREASES YOUR RISK OF
## CORONARY ARTERY DISEASE.

Weight training can reduce certain risk factors for coronary artery disease. Dr. Linn Goldberg of the University of Oregon Health Sciences Center studied the effect of weight training on fat buildup in the blood vessels. His participants trained three times per week for sixteen weeks. Results included a significant lowering of low-density lipoproteins (the "bad" cholesterol) and a reduction in total cholesterol levels.

Other studies also indicate that weight training, especially when combined with low-calorie dieting, can significantly reduce triglycerides, increase high-density lipoproteins (the "good" cholesterol), and lower the important risk factor of total cholesterol divided by high-density lipoproteins.

## MYTH:
## WEIGHT TRAINING IS
## DANGEROUS FOR PEOPLE WITH
## HIGH BLOOD PRESSURE.

Many earlier studies determined that isometric contractions elevated blood pressure to very high levels. Some people, including physicians, incorrectly assumed that weight training did the same. This is not the case.

Dr. Wayne Westcott, fitness advisor for the YMCA of the USA, studied the blood pressure responses of over one hundred subjects as they completed an eleven-exercise Nautilus circuit. He noted a small increase in systolic blood pressure and a small decrease in diastolic blood pressure, a perfectly normal response to rigorous exercise. He concluded that sensible weight training does not have an adverse affect on blood pressure in healthy adults. Dr. Westcott warned, however, that maximum lifts, breath-holding, isometric contractions, and hand-gripping can produce excessive blood pressure responses. Such activities should be avoided.

Researchers at Johns Hopkins University found that weight training can be a valuable method of lowering high blood pressure. They concluded that appropriate weight training is a very safe—but often neglected—mode of exercise for heart patients.

# MYTH:
# OLDER MEN SHOULD NOT ENGAGE IN WEIGHT TRAINING. THEY SHOULD WALK OR SWIM INSTEAD.

Even in your seventies, you can improve your strength level through proper weight training. In a University of Southern California study, a group of seventy-year-old men showed significant improvement in muscular strength following an eight-week weight-training program.

In the last ten years, I've personally trained several men over seventy who made remarkable strength gains during ten-week programs. Each man added three to six pounds of muscle to his physique. Added muscle contributes to any movement activity, and improves posture, elevates metabolism, and helps prevent injuries.

Weight training produces these benefits much more efficiently than does walking or swimming. Regardless of age, if a man can move, he can move against resistance and stimulate his muscles to grow.

# MYTH:
# IF SOMETHING HURTS DURING AN EXERCISE, STOP DOING IT.

There's productive pain during exercise, and there's destructive pain. The productive pain is a burning sensation in the muscle that usually occurs during the last repetition or two of an exercise. Super-slow, high-intensity exercise works a maximum percentage of the involved muscle's fibers, increasing demand for nutrient importation and waste exportation. This is accomplished by elevated blood volume to and from the muscle. The muscle swells and becomes engorged with intercellular fluid.

Engorgement of the involved muscles produces a dull, aching pain. The swelling muscle impinges various nerves and creates a burning sensation. Within minutes after termination of the exercise, the pain and burning dissipates as the engorgement diminishes. Such burning in the muscle should not cause concern. It merely indicates a highly effective exercise.

On the other hand, if you ever feel a sharp pain in the joint, *stop the exercise immediately*. Sharp joint pain can indicate injury to the joint and/or connective tissues. If the condition does not improve or worsens, see your personal physician.

## MYTH:
## WHATEVER MUSCLE YOU GAIN
## FROM WEIGHT TRAINING
## WILL TURN TO FAT ONCE YOU
## STOP EXERCISING.

Not true! Muscle is muscle, fat is fat, and there is no way to turn one into the other.

Muscle is 71 percent water, 22 percent proteins, and 7 percent lipids. Fat is 22 percent water, 6 percent proteins, and 72 percent lipids. Like apples and oranges, muscle and fat are genetically and chemically different.

When a man stops training, he seldom decreases his caloric intake. The result is a gradual decrease in the size and strength of his muscles and an increase in body fat stores. Since muscle and fat are so close to each other that they can intermingle, it appears that his muscles have turned to fat. Fortunately, muscle and fat levels don't change immediately when you stop exercising. You can work back to your previous level in a fraction of the time it took you to get there.

## MYTH:
## WEIGHT TRAINING WILL
## MAKE YOU LOOK LIKE
## ARNOLD SCHWARZENEGGER.

This is a double-edged myth. Many younger men involved with bodybuilding desperately want to look like Arnold. They read his articles and books, adhere to his routines, and eat his recommended foods and supplements. On the other hand, most middle-aged men do *not* want to look like Arnold. They find his muscularity unappealing, and they fear that weight training will overdevelop their muscles.

Both of these concepts are incorrect, and much of the reason centers around genetics. Genetics is an important factor in excelling in particular sports. For example, being tall improves your chances of being successful in professional basketball. For horse-racing jockeys, just the opposite is true. Your height can help or hurt you depending on the sport, but it's obvious that bouncing a basketball won't make you taller, nor will riding a horse make you shorter. Your height is primarily determined by genetics.

Champion bodybuilders are born with the genetic potential to develop excessively large muscles. Muscular potential, like height, can be judged quickly if you know what to look for. The length of your muscles—from the tendon attachment at one end to the tendon attachment at the other—is the most important factor in determining their potential size. The longer your muscles, the greater the cross-sectional area, and thus the greater the volume your muscles can reach.

A long muscle presumes above-average size in that muscle. A short muscle implies that the muscle will be below average in size. Both extremes are rare. Having extremely long or short muscles exclusively throughout your entire body is seldom seen. Approximately one man in a million has such genes.

Arnold Schwarzenegger is one of those men. He has very long muscles throughout his entire body. Woody Allen, on the other hand, is a prime example of someone born with short muscles. Frame size is less important than muscle length in determining your ultimate muscular mass.

The majority of people have muscles that are neither long nor short, but average. Average-length muscles produce average-sized muscles, even after years of training.

The length of your muscles is 100 percent genetic. You cannot change the length or size potential of your muscles, not through exercise, not through diet supplements, not through anything.

If you have long muscles, you're probably already stronger than other men your age—even if you've never trained. With properly applied weight training, your results will be significant and rapid. Gains in muscular size and strength will be several times faster for you than for the average trainee, whose gains will *always* be more difficult to produce.

Don't worry about looking, or not looking, like Arnold. Recognize your genetic potential, then maximize it in 32 days.

# =10=

# Measurements and Photographs

"I never knew how fat I was nor how flabby I looked," said one of the 32/32 participants, "until I evaluated my measurements and viewed my 'before' pictures."

## WARNING: DO NOT SKIP THE APPLICATION OF THIS CHAPTER

Take your measurements and photographs *before* you begin the 32/32 program. You'll be glad you did once the pounds and inches start melting away. You'll be able to see tangible differences when you compare your before-and-after results.

The objective of before-and-after measurements is to prompt you to record and recognize your present condition, motivate you to improve, help you to identify your achievements, and increase your knowledge of your body.

The most important quality of your measurements is their accuracy. You must follow the guidelines for making these measurements carefully. Be precise and consistent.

## SKINFOLD PINCH FOR FATNESS

Fatness and leanness are opposites. Fatness describes an abundance of body fat; leanness, a lack of body fat. Since most of your fat is stored

**37**

directly under the skin, measuring the thickness of pinched layers of skin and fat is a way to determine body fatness. Here's how to measure:

1. Have a friend do the measuring if possible, because you cannot pinch your own skinfold accurately.

2. Locate the first skinfold site on the back of your right upper arm (triceps area) midway between the shoulder and elbow. Let the arm hang loosely at the side.

3. Grasp a vertical fold of skin between the thumb and first finger. Pull the skin and fat away from the arm. The fold should not include any muscle, just skin and fat. Practice pinching and pulling the skin until no muscle is included.

4. Using a ruler, measure the thickness of the skinfold to the nearest quarter-inch by measuring the distance between the thumb and finger. Occasionally the top of the skinfold is thicker than the distance between the thumb and finger. To avoid this, keep the top of the skinfold level with the top of the thumb. Do not press the ruler against the skinfold, as this will flatten it out and make it appear thicker than it really is.

5. Take two separate measures of skinfold thickness, releasing the skin between each measure. Add them together and divide by two to determine the average thickness.

6. Locate the second skinfold site immediately adjacent to the right of the *umbilicus* or navel.

7. Grasp a vertical fold of skin between the thumb and first finger and follow the same technique as previously described.

8. Take two separate measurements of the abdominal skinfold thickness. Add them together and divide by two for an average.

9. Add the average triceps skinfold to the average abdominal skinfold. This is your combined total.

10. Estimate your percent body fat from the chart below.

| | |
|---|---|
| ³/₄ inch or less combined skinfold thickness | 5 – 9% |
| 1 inch combined skinfold thickness | 9 – 13% |
| 1 ¼ inches combined skinfold thickness | 13 – 18% |
| 1 ³/₄ inches combined skinfold thickness | 18 – 22% |
| Over 1³/₄ inches combined skinfold thickness | 27 – 32% |

Ideally, your combined skinfold thickness should be 1 inch or less. This means that your body fat level is below 13 percent, which is excellent. Within reason, the less fat you have under your skin and around your waist, the better off you are physically. By shrinking your skinfolds, your waist will automatically develop a tighter, more muscular appearance.

## 32/32 MEASUREMENTS

In addition to determining your present body fat, I suggest you keep records of the following before-and-after measurements.

1. Measure your weight and height. If possible, use a balance-type medical scale found in physicians' offices.

2. Take relaxed circumference measurements at nine sites: both upper arms midway between the elbow and the shoulder; chest at nipple level; three waist positions: 2 inches above the navel, at the navel, and 2 inches below the navel; hips; and both thighs just below the buttocks.

3. Determine total fat loss at the end of the program by multiplying percentage of body fat times body weight for the before-and-after tests. For example, if you weighed 200 pounds with 22 percent body fat at the start of the program, that's 44 pounds of fat. If you completed the program at 183 pounds and 13 percent body fat, that's 23.8 pounds of fat. The difference between 44 and 23.8 is 20.2 pounds of total fat loss.

4. Calculate the amount of muscle gained by subtracting the total weight lost from the total fat lost. In the example above, where fat loss equaled 20.2 pounds and weight loss equaled 17 pounds, 3.2 pounds of muscle were gained.

## 32/32
## BEFORE-AND-AFTER
## MEASUREMENTS

*9/20*

NAME _____*FRed Kieper*_____ AGE____*23*

DATE _____*7/5/94*_____ HEIGHT____*6'2"*

SKINFOLD

*Chest*

|  | Before | After | Difference |
|---|---|---|---|
| Triceps | *8* | *10* | _____ |
| Abdomen | *44* | *33* | _____ |
| *thigh* Total | *42* | *22* | _____ |
| *Total* Percentage | *94* | _____ | _____ |
| *Percentage* Fat pounds | _____ | _____ | _____ |

SCALE WEIGHT

|  | Before | After | Difference |
|---|---|---|---|
|  | *224* | _____ | _____ |

TOTAL FAT LOSS_____

MUSCLE GAINED_____

## CIRCUMFERENCE MEASUREMENTS

| | Before | After | Inches Lost |
|---|---|---|---|
| Right Arm | 13 1/2 | 13 1/2 | — |
| Left Arm | 13 | 13 1/4 | 1/4 |
| Chest | 42 1/2 | 41 1/2 | 1 |
| Waist: 2" above navel | 37 | 35 | 2 |
| Waist at navel | 39 1/4 | 37 1/2 | 2 |
| Waist: 2" below navel | 39 | 37 1/2 | 2 |
| Hips | 44 1/2 | | |
| Right Thigh | 25 | 24 1/2 | 1/2 |
| Left Thigh | 25 | 25 | — |

TOTAL INCHES LOST_____

## BEFORE-AND-AFTER
## PHOTOGRAPHS

It is important to have photographs taken of yourself in a tight bathing suit—like the ones shown in this book—before and after the 32-day program. It takes a little time and effort, but is well worth it.

Here are the guidelines you'll need to follow:

1.  Have your photographer use a 35-millimeter camera, if possible, loaded with black-and-white print film. He should turn the camera sideways for a vertical format negative.

2.  Wear a snug bathing suit (a solid color is best), and stand against an uncluttered, light background.

3.  Have the photographer move away from you until he can see your entire body in the viewfinder. He should sit in a chair and hold the camera level with your navel, preferably mounting the camera at this level on a tripod.

4.  Pose in three directions: front, side, and back, with your hands on top of your head in each shot and feet spaced evenly.

5.  Repeat the photo session in 32 days, wearing the same bathing suit and assuming identical poses.

6.  Instruct the photo processor to make your after prints exactly the same size as your before prints. *Important:* your height in all the before-and-after photos must be standardized for valid comparisons to be made and fat losses noted. This is done by comparison cropping at the processing lab.

## THE BOTTOM LINE

Measurements and evaluations can be both meaningful and confusing, but the bottom line is:

- **if you have more than 1/2 inch of fat (skinfold thickness) beside your navel,**

or

- if your waist is significantly larger than 32 inches,

  then

  you are a prime candidate for the 32/32 program!

# –=11=–
# What 32/32 Men Accomplished

Committing yourself to a rigorous training program like 32/32 requires unremitting determination. Ditto for adhering to a descending-calorie diet. High-intensity, super-slow exercise is grueling. Counting calories is not much fun either.

"I was in the locker room after a hard workout," said one trainee, "when I muttered to no one in particular, 'is it all worth it?' An older man, about 65, looked over and responded, 'When you go to the doctor and he tells you that your fat percentage, cholesterol level, and blood pressure are normal, then it's all worth it.'"

The response made an indelible impression.

"I instantly matured in my reasoning for putting out this effort," the trainee, then in his mid-twenties, recalled.

The two men relied on different motivations, the elder on health, the younger on looks and sexual appeal. Your motivation in your thirties to fifties is likely to be a combination of these.

If you're just getting involved in an exercise program after a long period of inactivity, it'll be a challenge to summon the discipline required. "Not again today," your body will seem to say. "I'm comfortable as I am—leave me alone!"

Or your taste buds may tingle for the chocolate chip cookies you see on television. "What's it going to hurt?" you ask. "I'll make up for it by skipping breakfast tomorrow."

You need motivation to cut back on calories, start exercising intensely, and control certain risk factors. The following men exemplify motivation in action.

**"**Since going through the program, I'm much more aware of my eating behavior. My new waistline is a constant reminder and influences my menu choices, especially when I'm dining out.**"**

### MICHAEL BROWN
### age 42

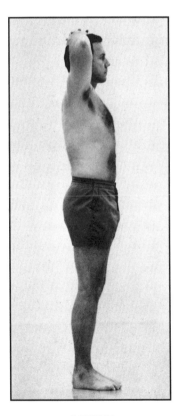

Lost
24½
pounds
of fat

Built
5¼
pounds
of muscle

AND
TRIMMED
3¾
inches off
his waist

in
32 days!

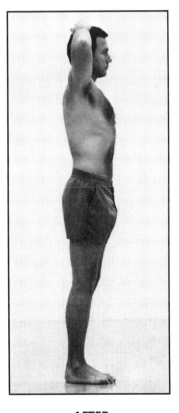

**BEFORE**
Waist Size:
38½

**AFTER**
Waist Size:
34¾

*"*My posture has improved dramatically.
I now sit tall, stand tall, and feel tall.*"*

**RON TRAVIS**
**age 46**

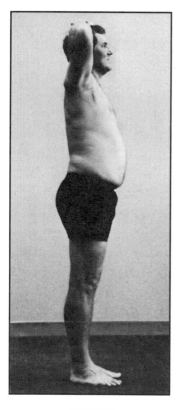

Lost
21¾
pounds
of fat

Built
5
pounds
of muscle

AND
TRIMMED
3⅝
inches off
his waist

in
32 days!

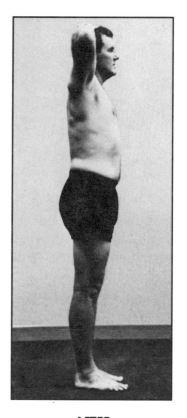

**BEFORE**
Waist Size:
39⅝

**AFTER**
Waist Size:
36

"I was in fairly good condition when I started and felt if I dropped 10 pounds and 3 percent body fat, I would be satisfied. I exceeded these goals and improved areas of my body that I've never been able to zero in on. I've never seen such dramatic and positive results in just 32 days."

## RALPH GOODMAN
### age 48

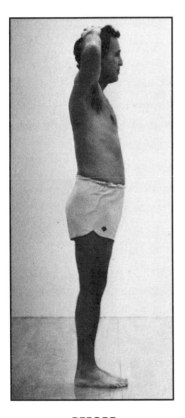

Lost
17
pounds
of fat

Built
2³/4
pounds
of muscle

AND
TRIMMED
2³/4
inches off
his waist

in
32 days!

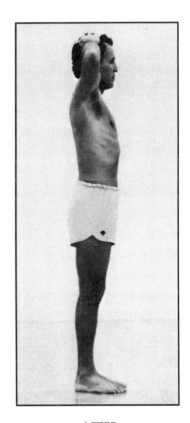

| BEFORE | AFTER |
|---|---|
| Waist Size: | Waist Size: |
| 33¼ | 30½ |

"My posture has improved, I have more energy, and I have a much greater appreciation for combining strength-building exercise with diet."

### RICHARD IVES
**age 47**

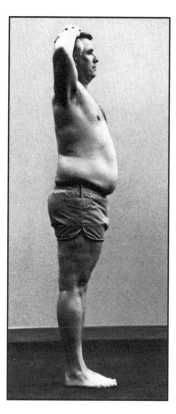

Lost
24³/₄
pounds
of fat

Built
4
pounds
of muscle

AND
TRIMMED
6
inches off
his waist

in
32 days!

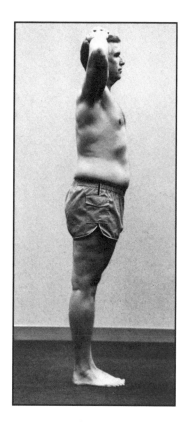

**BEFORE**
Waist Size:
45

**AFTER**
Waist Size:
39

**"**This has definitely opened my eyes to a better way of eating and exercising. Many thanks for starting me on a much healthier road to longer living.**"**

### KEN R. OAKES
#### age 38

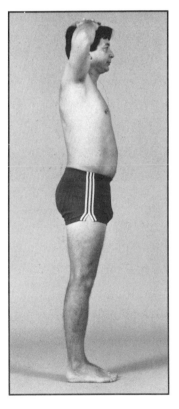

Lost
17
pounds
of fat

Built
4¹/₄
pounds
of muscle

AND
TRIMMED
2⁵/₈
inches off
his waist

in
32 days!

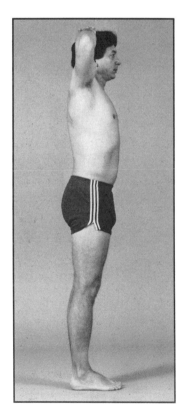

**BEFORE**
Waist Size:
36⁵/₈

**AFTER**
Waist Size:
34

*"*I feel better physically and mentally. I also feel better about myself and my relationship with my wife and family.*"*

### MICHAEL J. HENTZ
### age 36

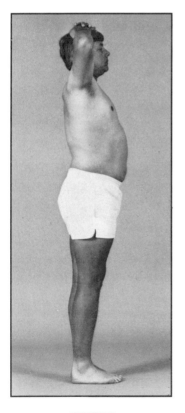

Lost
22³/₄
pounds of
fat

Built
3
pounds
of muscle

AND
TRIMMED
5¹/₂
inches off
his waist

in
32 days!

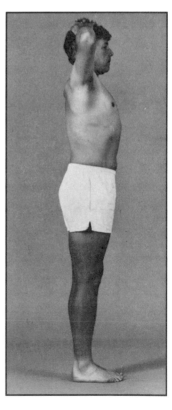

**BEFORE**
Waist Size:
42¹/₂

**AFTER**
Waist Size:
37

# —=12=—
# Before Getting Started

There are a number of steps involved in starting the 32/32 program.

## GET YOUR DOCTOR'S PERMISSION.

Before you begin this program, be sure your doctor knows you plan to modify both your eating and exercising habits. Show him this book so he knows what is involved. He'll likely recommend a thorough physical examination if he hasn't given you one in the last year.

There are a few people I feel should *not* try this 32/32 program: children and teenagers; men with certain types of heart, liver, or kidney disease; diabetics; and those suffering from some types of arthritis. This should not be taken as an all-inclusive list. Some men should follow the 32/32 course only with their physician's specific guidance and recommendations. Consult your doctor beforehand to play it safe.

## DO YOUR "BEFORE" MEASUREMENTS AND PHOTOGRAPHS.

Don't procrastinate on taking your measurements and photographs. Without accurate assessments, you'll be traveling a difficult road without a good support system. For maximum effectiveness, 32/32 should be followed step-by-step.

## ✕ BUY FOOD MEASURING SPOONS, CUPS, AND A SMALL SCALE.

Most people overestimate one-half cup of orange juice, one tablespoon of raisins, or one ounce of mozzarella cheese. Such practices lead to sloppy recipe preparation, inaccurate calorie counting, and inefficient fat loss. It is important to become familiar with and correctly use measuring spoons, cups, and food scales.

All of these items can be purchased inexpensively at your local department store or supermarket. With food scales, however, you'd be well advised to spend more money to purchase a battery-operated, digital scale instead of the less-expensive, spring-loaded type.

## ✕ TAKE A VITAMIN-MINERAL TABLET EACH DAY.

Although the 32/32 diet is well balanced, you should take *one* multiple vitamin-with-minerals tablet each morning. Be certain no nutrient listed on the label exceeds 100 percent of the U.S. Recommended Daily Allowances. High-potency supplements are a waste of money.

## EXAMINE THE 32/32 MENUS, RECIPES, AND SHOPPING LISTS.

Glance through the 32/32 menus, recipes, and shopping lists (Chapters 13 through 16) for an overview of what you'll be eating during the next month. Your results will be more effective if you plan ahead.

## KEEP FOOD SUBSTITUTIONS TO A MINIMUM.

I recommend that you follow the menus and recipes exactly as indicated. The 32/32 participants who obtain the best results almost never vary from the listed foods. But I know there are times when some men must make substitutions for certain foods. For example, those of you who are allergic to milk may substitute one ounce of cheese or one cup of low-fat yogurt for one cup of milk in any menu. And those who are vegetarians may exchange one egg or a cup of cooked dried beans or peas for one meat serving.

Those fond of frozen dinners are in luck. In the troubleshooting section (Chapter 17), three Lean Cuisine frozen dinners and eight other frozen dinners with the acceptable proportion of carbohydrates, fats, and proteins are listed as substitutions for any evening meal. Do not, however, use the frozen dinners more than four times per week.

## CONSIDER GIVING UP ALCOHOL DURING THE PROGRAM.

If possible, give up alcoholic drinks entirely until you have reached your fat-loss goal. If you feel you must have a drink, limit your consumption to one light beer no more than three times per week. You'll see a light beer mentioned as an optional snack on some of the menus.

Most men completing 32/32 found that one light beer didn't seem satisfying compared to their previous drinking habits. My advice to you is the same advice I gave to them: *avoid alcohol during the program*. Stick to more nutritious snacks to synergize your results.

## HAVE A PARTNER GO THROUGH THE PROGRAM WITH YOU.

You'll probably obtain better fat-loss and muscle-building results if you  go through the program with an out-of-shape friend. Here are the guidelines for choosing a partner.

1.  Your partner should be overfat to a similar degree. He should have eating and exercising habits resembling your own.

2.  Your partner needs to be interested in losing fat and getting in shape to the point of making a serious 32-day commitment. That commitment means you'll be exercising together for at least one hour, three times per week. Each of your joint training sessions should take approximately forty minutes, including twenty minutes spent supervising your partner's workout.

3.  Your partner should be someone you won't feel pressured to impress, but a person you feel close to and can be honest with.

4.  Your partner should not be a person who judges and criticizes you or offers nonconstructive advice.

5.  Your partner needs to be available for daily phone calls, three-times-a-week workouts, and possible meetings during times of weakening resolve.

6.  Your partner *should not* be your spouse, parent, or other family member. Normal interpersonal problems may interfere with your program.

Once you have a candidate, it is important to explain exactly how you want to be treated: strictly or loosely. Go over responsibilities and the roles you expect each other to fulfill. These include punctuality, weighing in, recording your workouts on cards, reinforcing positive behaviors, and understanding and sharing your problems.

## DRINK PLENTY OF
## COLD WATER EACH DAY.

Invariably, the men who lose the most fat in 32 days have the highest daily water intakes. Mark Sandberg, who lost over 25 pounds of fat in 32 days, drank two gallons of water a day during the last weeks of the program. Ken Howell, who went through the program three times and lost 36¼ pounds of fat, consumed from one to two gallons of water each day for over two months.

Water is one of the most important catalysts in losing fat, and in keeping it off. Here's why:

*   Water suppresses your appetite and helps your system metabolize stored fat. A gallon of ice-cold water (40 degrees Fahrenheit) requires approximately 200 calories of energy to warm it to core body temperature (98.6 degrees Fahrenheit). Spread that gallon of water out over six to eight hours and your body requires even more heat energy to warm it.

*   Water in large amounts is the best solution for fluid retention.

- Water is important in the muscle-building process, since skeletal muscles are over 70 percent water.

- Water helps prevent the sagging skin that often follows significant fat loss. Water plumps the skin and leaves it clear, healthy, and resilient.

- Water helps flush the body of waste materials.

- Water helps relieve constipation.

If you want to lose fat more efficiently, gradually drink more water each day. Begin with eight 8-ounce glasses, or two quarts, of cold water each day for the first week. Increase this by one glass per day until you get to sixteen 8-ounce glasses, or one gallon a day. Then, you may want to work up to two gallons a day. By that time, if you've followed the diet and exercise program as well, you should be lean, strong, and healthy.

If you can't imagine drinking so much plain water, you might try other beverages which are over 99 percent water: artificially flavored carbonated water, mineral water, diet soda, coffee, and tea. Naturally, the cost of these drinks is much higher. Carefully read the labels to make sure that the beverages you consume in place of water contain 0 to 1 calorie per serving. If you are sensitive to caffeine, sodium, or aspartame, make sure that it is *not* included on the contents listing.

## AVOID INTENSE ACTIVITY ON YOUR NON-EXERCISE DAYS.

Too much activity can be more harmful to your body than too little activity, especially when you're following a low-calorie diet. If you exercise intensely more than three times per week, your system soon reaches a state of overtraining. Fat losses and strength gains slow rather than accelerate. You eventually get the blahs, have little enthusiasm, and break your diet. At this point you are close to "burning the candle at both ends, and trying to light it in the middle too."

During your participation in the 32/32 diet and exercise program, it is to your advantage to keep your outside activities to a minimum. Naturally, you can continue with your normal work and household responsibilities. Simply avoid vigorous activities such as running, skiing, racquetball, and basketball. Light recreational activities not carried to extremes are fine.

Once you reach your fat-loss goal, you can get involved in various strenuous sports and fitness activities if you wish.

## START THE 32/32 DIET ON
## THE FIRST DAY OF THE MONTH.

Although this is the last and least important recommendation in this chapter, I've found that the regimen is easier for most men to follow if the days of the diet correspond with the days of the month. In other words, if you begin this diet on May 1, then Day 1 and May 1 have the same numbers; and the perfect synchronization continues until the last one or two days.

## THE NEXT STEP

Review this chapter again, act on the salient requirements, and prepare to begin the 32/32 plan.

# _=13=_
# 32/32 Diet: Days 1-16

The menus and recipes in the 32/32 diet are designed for maximum fat-loss effectiveness and nutritional value. For best results, follow them exactly.

The calories you consume each day will gradually descend from 1,500 for Days 1-16, to 1,400 for Days 17-32. This type of descending-calorie eating plan is the most scientifically productive way to lose fat.

Each day you will choose from a limited selection of foods for breakfast and lunch. I've found that most men can consume the same basic breakfast and the same basic lunch for months with little or no modification. Ample variety during your evening meal, however, will make daily eating interesting and enjoyable. Additionally, the 32/32 diet includes a mid-afternoon and a late-night snack to keep your energy high and your hunger low.

Most of the recipes used with the evening meals yield two servings. Making two servings allows you to freeze one portion for the following week. If you'd rather prepare only one serving, simply cut the ingredients in half.

Begin Day 1 on the first day of the month and continue as directed for eight days. Days 9-16 are an exact repeat of Days 1-8. The menus for Days 17-32 are in the next chapter.

The calorie content of each food is noted in parentheses. An asterisk (*) preceding a listing indicates that a recipe for that dish is given in Chapter 15.

Chapter 16 contains the shopping lists for all your groceries.

# Day 1 & Day 9

**Total calories, including snacks: 1,501**

### BREAKFAST: 307 CALORIES

BASIC BREAKFAST ONE
Cereal choices (1-ounce size, 110 calories)
• Nabisco Shredded Wheat
• Kellogg's Frosted Mini Wheats
• Kellogg's NutriGrain Wheat or Corn
• Post Grape Nuts
• Ralston Purina Almond Delight
• Ralston Purina Sun Flakes Crispy Wheat & Rice
• ³/₄ cup cooked oatmeal, sprinkled with
   cinnamon and low-calorie sweetener
• Quaker Oat Bran: one serving of oat bran (90)
   sprinkled with one tablespoon raisins (25)
¹/₂ cup skim milk (45)
¹/₂ cup orange juice (55)
2 slices reduced-calorie bread, toasted (80)
1 teaspoon low-calorie margarine (17)
Noncaloric beverage
**OR**
BASIC BREAKFAST TWO
* Tropical Breakfast Shake, Recipe #1 (267)
1 slice reduced-calorie bread, toasted (40)

### LUNCH: 399 CALORIES

BASIC LUNCH
Roast Beef, Tuna or Turkey Sandwich:
   2 slices reduced-calorie bread (80)
   ¹/₂ tablespoon low-calorie mayonnaise (20)
   2 slices tomato (14)
   1 lettuce leaf (2)
   1 ounce low-calorie cheese (1¹/₂ slices) (50)
   2 ounces lean sliced roast beef (from the deli)
   **OR** ¹/₂ can (6¹/₂-oz. size) water-packed tuna (110)
   **OR** 2 ounces roasted turkey
1 cup skim milk (90)
²/₃ cup one of the following:
• Blueberries (33)
• Strawberries, sliced (33)
• Cantaloupe, diced (33)
• ¹/₃ cup unsweetened applesauce (33)

### SNACK: 155 CALORIES

1 whole graham cracker (4 sections) (60)
1 cup hot tea or coffee (0)
1 tablespoon peanut butter (95)*
**OR**
1 cup low-sodium bouillon (12)
4 saltines (48)
1 tablespoon peanut butter (95)*

* OPTION: If desired, omit peanut butter
  for a light beer at evening snack.

### DINNER: 498 CALORIES

* Mandarin Chicken, Recipe #2 (315)
1 small potato (2½-inch diameter,
  4½ ounces), baked (90)
SALAD:
   1 cup chopped lettuce (9)
   3 slices tomato (21)
   1 tablespoon diet Italian dressing (6)
1 slice reduced-calorie bread (40)
1 teaspoon low-calorie margarine (17)
Noncaloric beverage

### SNACK: 142 CALORIES

½ cup ice milk (100)
¾ cup strawberries (fresh or frozen) (42)

* OPTION: Light beer (95) (if peanut butter was
  omitted from afternoon snack)

# Day 2 & Day 10

**Total calories including snacks: 1,495**

### BREAKFAST: 307 CALORIES

BASIC BREAKFAST ONE **OR**
BASIC BREAKFAST TWO

### LUNCH: 399 CALORIES

BASIC LUNCH

### SNACK: 155 CALORIES

1 whole graham cracker (4 sections) (60)
1 cup hot tea or coffee (0)
1 tablespoon peanut butter (95)
**OR**
1 cup low-sodium bouillon (12)
4 saltines (48)
1 tablespoon peanut butter (95)

### DINNER: 494 CALORIES

* Vegetable-Topped Fish Fillet, Recipe #3 (235)
* Waldorf Special, Recipe #4 (129)
1 slice reduced-calorie bread (40)
1 cup skim milk (90)
Noncaloric beverage

### SNACK: 140 CALORIES

2 cups packaged microwave popcorn (140)
**OR**
1 tablespoon popcorn popped in 1 tablespoon
   vegetable oil (140)
Noncaloric beverage

# Day 3 & Day 11

Total calories including snacks: 1,500

**BREAKFAST: 307 CALORIES**

BASIC BREAKFAST ONE **OR**
BASIC BREAKFAST TWO

**LUNCH: 399 CALORIES**

BASIC LUNCH

**SNACK: 155 CALORIES**

1 whole graham cracker (4 sections) (60)
1 cup hot tea or coffee (0)
1 tablespoon peanut butter (95)
**OR**
1 cup low-sodium bouillon (12)
4 saltines (48)
1 tablespoon peanut butter (95)

**DINNER: 493 CALORIES**

* Cheesy Macaroni, Recipe #5 (390)
SALAD:
      1 cup fresh young spinach leaves (9)
      5 fresh mushrooms, sliced (5)
      1 tablespoon diet Italian dressing (6)
1 slice reduced-calorie bread (40)
1 teaspoon low-calorie margarine (17)
1/2 cup strawberries, sliced (25)
Noncaloric beverage

**SNACK: 146 CALORIES**

1 medium peach (6 ounces, 2³/₄-inch diameter)
**OR**
1/2 cup canned peaches, juice-packed (50),
      topped with 1/2 cup vanilla low-fat yogurt
      (66) and 1/2 graham cracker (2 sections) (30)

# Day 4 & Day 12

### Total calories including snacks: 1,492

### BREAKFAST: 307 CALORIES

BASIC BREAKFAST ONE **OR**
BASIC BREAKFAST TWO

### LUNCH: 399 CALORIES

BASIC LUNCH

### SNACK: 155 CALORIES

1 whole graham cracker (4 sections) (60)
1 cup hot tea or coffee (0)
1 tablespoon peanut butter (95)*
**OR**
1 cup low-sodium bouillon (12)
4 saltines (48)
1 tablespoon peanut butter (95)*

* OPTION: Omit peanut butter for light
  beer at evening snack.

### DINNER: 489 CALORIES

* Lean sirloin, broiled, 3 ounces (176), topped with
  Peppers 'n' Onions, Recipe #6 (40)
1 ear corn (5 inches long), boiled (70)
1 teaspoon low-calorie margarine (17)
1 cup French-style green beans, steamed (31)
SALAD:
    1/2 banana (medium), sliced (50)
    1 tablespoon raisins (25)
    1 teaspoon low-calorie mayonnaise (13),
    served on 1 lettuce leaf (2)
1 slice reduced-calorie bread (40)
1/2 tablespoon low-calorie margarine (25)
Noncaloric beverage

### SNACK: 150 CALORIES

Remaining 1/2 banana, sliced (50)**
1/2 cup strawberries, sliced (25)
1 1/4 graham cracker (5 sections) (75)
Noncaloric beverage

**OPTION: If having beer at evening snack,
  have banana with afternoon snack.

# Day 5 & Day 13

**Total calories including snacks: 1,496**

### BREAKFAST: 307 CALORIES

BASIC BREAKFAST ONE **OR**
BASIC BREAKFAST TWO

### LUNCH: 399 CALORIES

BASIC LUNCH

### SNACK: 155 CALORIES

1 whole graham cracker (4 sections) (60)
1 cup hot tea or coffee (0)
1 tablespoon peanut butter (95)
**OR**
1 cup low-sodium bouillon (12)
4 saltines (48)
1 tablespoon peanut butter (95)

### DINNER: 490 CALORIES

* Chicken Pea Bake, Recipe #7 (216)
1 small potato (2½-inch diameter,
   4½ ounces), baked (90),
   topped with 2 tablespoons plain
   low-fat yogurt (19)
SALAD:
      1 cup chopped lettuce (9)
      1 small stalk celery (4 inches long), chopped (3)
      2 tablespoons grated carrot (6)
      2 slices tomato, chopped (14)
      1 tablespoon diet Italian dressing (6)
1 slice reduced-calorie bread (40)
1 teaspoon low-calorie margarine (17)
2 slices pineapple, juice-packed (70)
Noncaloric beverage

### SNACK: 145 CALORIES

½ cup ice milk (100)
¾ graham cracker (3 sections) (45)

# Day 6 & Day 14

### Total calories including snacks: 1,499

### BREAKFAST: 307 CALORIES

BASIC BREAKFAST ONE **OR**
BASIC BREAKFAST TWO

### LUNCH: 399 CALORIES

BASIC LUNCH

### SNACK: 155 CALORIES

1 whole graham cracker (4 sections) (60)
1 cup hot tea or coffee (0)
1 tablespoon peanut butter (95)*
**OR**
1 cup low-sodium bouillon (12)
4 saltines (48)
1 tablespoon peanut butter (95)*

\* OPTION: Omit peanut butter for
light beer at evening snack.

### DINNER: 495 CALORIES

\* Apple Chops, Recipe #8 (254)
3/4 cup French-style green beans, steamed (23)
1 sweet potato (5 inches long, 2-inch diameter) (161)
1 teaspoon low-calorie margarine (17)
1 slice reduced-calorie bread (40)
Noncaloric beverage

### SNACK: 143 CALORIES

1 ounce part-skim mozzarella cheese (90)**
1½ slices pineapple, juice-packed (53)
Noncaloric beverage

\*\*OPTION: If having light beer
at evening snack, have mozzarella
cheese with afternoon snack.

# Day 7 & Day 15

### Total calories including snacks: 1,542

**BREAKFAST: 307 CALORIES**

> BASIC BREAKFAST ONE **OR**
> BASIC BREAKFAST TWO

**LUNCH: 399 CALORIES**

> BASIC LUNCH

**SNACK: 155 CALORIES**

> 1 whole graham cracker (4 sections) (60)
> 1 cup hot tea or coffee (0)
> 1 tablespoon peanut butter (95)
> **OR**
> 1 cup low-sodium bouillon (12)
> 4 saltines (48)
> 1 tablespoon peanut butter (95)

**DINNER: 526 CALORIES**

> * Quick & Easy Lasagna, Recipe #9 (356)
> 1 cup chopped broccoli, steamed (40)
> 2 slices reduced-calorie bread (80)
> 1/2 cup unsweetened applesauce (50)
> Noncaloric beverage

**SNACK: 155 CALORIES**

> 1/2 cup ice milk (100)
> 1/2 cup strawberries, sliced (25)
> 1/2 graham cracker (2 sections) (30)

# Day 8 & Day 16

### Total calories including snacks: 1,496

### BREAKFAST: 307 CALORIES

BASIC BREAKFAST ONE **OR**
BASIC BREAKFAST TWO

### LUNCH: 399 CALORIES

BASIC LUNCH

### SNACK: 155 CALORIES

1 whole graham cracker (4 sections) (60)
1 cup hot tea or coffee (0)
1 tablespoon peanut butter (95)
**OR**
1 cup low-sodium bouillon (12)
4 saltines (48)
1 tablespoon peanut butter (95)

### DINNER: 495 CALORIES

\* Sweet 'n' Sour Meatballs, Recipe #10 (298)
1/2 cup white rice (90)
1/2 cup unsweetened applesauce (50),
    sprinkled with cinnamon
1 slice reduced-calorie bread (40)
1 teaspoon low-calorie margarine (17)
Noncaloric beverage

### SNACK: 140 CALORIES

1 ounce part-skim mozzarella cheese (90)
1 small apple (50)

# —=14=—
# 32/32 Diet: Days 17–32

Begin Day 17 on the seventeenth day of the month and continue as directed for eight days.

Days 25-32 are an exact repeat of Days 17-24.

Approximately 100 calories daily have been deducted from each of the previous sixteen days' menus. For the second part of the 32/32 eating plan, pay close attention to the changes in the afternoon and evening snacks.

Basic Breakfasts One and Two, and Basic Lunch are identical to those during Days 1–16.

One change is that an apple (average size, with skin) replaces peanut butter in the snack that includes the graham cracker and tea or coffee.

Calories for each food are noted in parentheses. An asterisk (*) preceding a listing indicates that a recipe for that dish is given in Chapter 15.

The recipes are identical to those you followed the first sixteen days, with the addition of three alternate dinner menus. For variety, any of the new dinner menus may be substituted for any of the previous eight dinner menus.

A shopping list that includes items contained in the alternate dinners is included in Chapter 16.

You are halfway through the program, twice as close to your goals and growing strong!

# Day 17 & Day 25

### Total calories including snacks: 1,394

### BREAKFAST: 307 CALORIES

BASIC BREAKFAST ONE **OR**
BASIC BREAKFAST TWO

### LUNCH: 399 CALORIES

BASIC LUNCH

### SNACK: 140 CALORIES

³/₄ graham cracker (3 sections) (45)
1 cup hot tea or coffee (0)
1 apple (3-inch diameter) (95)*
**OR**
1 cup low-sodium bouillon (12)
3 saltines (36)
1 tablespoon peanut butter (95)*

* OPTION: Omit apple or peanut butter for a
  light beer at evening snack.

### DINNER: 498 CALORIES

* Mandarin Chicken, Recipe #2 (315)
1 small potato (2¹/₂-inch diameter, 4¹/₂ ounces),
  baked (90)
SALAD:
    1 cup chopped lettuce (9)
    3 slices tomato (21)
    1 tablespoon diet Italian dressing (6)
1 slice reduced-calorie bread (40)
1 teaspoon low-calorie margarine (17)
Noncaloric beverage

### SNACK: 50 CALORIES

2 tablespoons raisins (50)

* OPTION: Light beer (95) if apple or peanut
  butter omitted from afternoon snack.

# Day 18 & Day 26

### Total calories including snacks: 1,404

**BREAKFAST: 307 CALORIES**

BASIC BREAKFAST ONE **OR**
BASIC BREAKFAST TWO

**LUNCH: 399 CALORIES**

BASIC LUNCH

**SNACK: 140 CALORIES**

3/4 graham cracker (3 sections) (45)
1 cup hot tea or coffee (0)
1 apple (3-inch diameter) (95)
**OR**
1 cup low-sodium bouillon (12)
3 saltines (36)
1 tablespoon peanut butter (95)

**DINNER: 494 CALORIES**

* Vegetable-Topped Fish Fillet, Recipe #3 (235)
* Waldorf Special, Recipe #4 (129)
1 slice reduced-calorie bread (40)
1 cup skim milk (90)
Noncaloric beverage

**SNACK: 64 CALORIES**

1/2 cup sliced banana, frozen (64)
  Slice and wrap in aluminum foil, then freeze.
  Let thaw approximately 5 minutes before eating.

# Day 19 & Day 27

**Total calories including snacks: 1,391**

### BREAKFAST: 307 CALORIES

BASIC BREAKFAST ONE **OR**
BASIC BREAKFAST TWO

### LUNCH: 399 CALORIES

BASIC LUNCH

### SNACK: 140 CALORIES

3/4 graham cracker (3 sections) (45)
1 cup hot tea or coffee (0)
1 apple (3-inch diameter) (95)
**OR**
1 cup low-sodium bouillon (12)
3 saltines (36)
1 tablespoon peanut butter (95)

### DINNER: 492 CALORIES

\* Cheesy Macaroni, Recipe #5 (390)
SALAD:
    1 cup fresh young spinach leaves (9)
    5 fresh mushrooms, sliced (5)
    1 tablespoon diet Italian dressing (6)
1 slice reduced-calorie bread (40)
1 teaspoon low-calorie margarine (17)
1/2 cup strawberries, sliced (25)
Noncaloric beverage

### SNACK: 53 CALORIES

1 1/2 slices pineapple, juice-packed (53)
**OR**
2 tablespoons raisins (50)
1 cup hot tea or coffee (0)

# Day 20 & Day 28

**Total calories including snacks: 1,377**

### BREAKFAST: 307 CALORIES

BASIC BREAKFAST ONE **OR**
BASIC BREAKFAST TWO

### LUNCH: 399 CALORIES

BASIC LUNCH

### SNACK: 140 CALORIES

3/4 graham cracker (3 sections) (45)
1 cup hot tea or coffee (0)
1 apple (3-inch diameter) (95)*
**OR**
1 cup low-sodium bouillon (12)
3 saltines (36)
1 tablespoon peanut butter (95)*

* OPTION: Omit apple or peanut butter for
light beer at evening snack.

### DINNER: 481 CALORIES

* Lean sirloin, broiled, 3 ounces (176), topped with
Peppers 'n' Onions, Recipe #6 (40)
1 ear corn (5 inches long), boiled (70)
1 teaspoon low-calorie margarine (17)
1 cup French-style green beans, steamed (31)
SALAD:
1/2 banana (medium), sliced (50)
1 tablespoon raisins (25)
1 teaspoon low-calorie mayonnaise (13),
served on 1 lettuce leaf (2)
1 slice reduced-calorie bread (40)
1 teaspoon low-calorie margarine (17)
Noncaloric beverage

### SNACK: 50 CALORIES

1 medium peach (6 ounces, 23/4-inch diameter) (50)**
**OR**
1/2 cup canned peaches, juice-packed (50)**

**OPTION: If having light beer as evening snack,
have peach with afternoon snack.

# Day 21 & Day 29

### Total calories including snacks: 1,400

**BREAKFAST:** 307 CALORIES

BASIC BREAKFAST ONE **OR**
BASIC BREAKFAST TWO

**LUNCH:** 399 CALORIES

BASIC LUNCH

**SNACK:** 140 CALORIES

3/4 graham cracker (3 sections) (45)
1 cup hot tea or coffee (0)
1 apple (3-inch diameter) (95)
**OR**
1 cup low-sodium bouillon (12)
3 saltines (36)
1 tablespoon peanut butter (95)

**DINNER:** 490 CALORIES

* Chicken Pea Bake, Recipe #7 (216)
1 small potato (2¹/₂-inch diameter,
    4¹/₂ ounces), baked (90)
    topped with 2 tablespoons plain
    low-fat yogurt (19)
SALAD:
        1 cup chopped lettuce (9)
        1 small stalk celery (4 inches long), chopped (3)
        2 tablespoons grated carrot (6)
        2 slices tomato, chopped (14)
        1 tablespoon diet Italian dressing (6)
1 slice reduced-calorie bread (40)
1 teaspoon low-calorie margarine (17)
2 slices pineapple, juice-packed (70)
Noncaloric beverage

**SNACK:** 64 CALORIES

¹/₂ cup sliced banana (64)
    Slice and wrap in aluminum foil, then freeze.
    Let thaw approximately 5 minutes before eating.

# Day 22 & Day 30

### Total calories including snacks: 1,394

## BREAKFAST: 307 CALORIES

BASIC BREAKFAST ONE **OR**
BASIC BREAKFAST TWO

## LUNCH: 399 CALORIES

BASIC LUNCH

## SNACK: 140 CALORIES

³/₄ graham cracker (3 sections) (45)
1 cup hot tea or coffee (0)
1 apple (3-inch diameter) (95)*
**OR**
1 cup low-sodium bouillon (12)
3 saltines (36)
1 tablespoon peanut butter (95)*

*OPTION: Omit peanut butter for light
    beer at evening snack.

## DINNER: 495 CALORIES

* Apple Chops, Recipe #8 (254)
³/₄ cup French-style green beans, steamed (23)
1 sweet potato (5 inches long, 2-inch diameter (161)
1 teaspoon low-calorie margarine (17)
1 slice reduced-calorie bread (40)
Noncaloric beverage

## SNACK: 53 CALORIES

1¹/₂ slices pineapple, juice-packed (53)**
Noncaloric beverage

**OPTION: If having light beer at evening snack,
    have pineapple with afternoon snack.

# Day 23 & Day 31

**Total calories including snacks: 1,422**

## BREAKFAST: 307 CALORIES

BASIC BREAKFAST ONE **OR**
BASIC BREAKFAST TWO

## LUNCH: 399 CALORIES

BASIC LUNCH

## SNACK: 140 CALORIES

3/4 graham cracker (3 sections) (45)
1 cup hot tea or coffee (0)
1 apple (3-inch diameter) (95)
**OR**
1 cup low-sodium bouillon (12)
3 saltines (36)
1 tablespoon peanut butter (95)

## DINNER: 491 CALORIES

* Quick & Easy Lasagna, Recipe #9 (356)
1 cup chopped broccoli, steamed (40)
2 slices reduced-calorie bread (80)
1/2 cup unsweetened applesauce (50)
Noncaloric beverage

## SNACK: 50 CALORIES

1 medium peach (6 ounces, 23/4-inch diameter) (50)
**OR**
1/2 cup canned peaches, juice-packed (50)

# Day 24 & Day 32

**Total calories including snacks: 1,405**

## BREAKFAST: 307 CALORIES

BASIC BREAKFAST ONE **OR**
BASIC BREAKFAST TWO

## LUNCH: 399 CALORIES

BASIC LUNCH

## SNACK: 140 CALORIES

3/4 graham cracker (3 sections) (45)
1 cup hot tea or coffee (0)
1 apple (3-inch diameter) (95)
**OR**
1 cup low-sodium bouillon (12)
3 saltines (36)
1 tablespoon peanut butter (95)

## DINNER: 495 CALORIES

* Sweet 'n' Sour Meatballs, Recipe #10 (298)
1/2 cup white rice (90)
1/2 cup unsweetened applesauce (50),
    sprinkled with cinnamon
1 slice reduced-calorie bread (40)
1 teaspoon low-calorie margarine (17)
Noncaloric beverage

## SNACK: 64 CALORIES

1/2 cup sliced banana, frozen (64)

# ALTERNATE DINNER MENUS

For variety, substitute any of the following
for any of the dinner menus:

### ALTERNATE
### DINNER MENU A: 496 CALORIES

* Huevos Rancheros, Recipe #11 (272)
* Spanish Rice, Recipe #12 (159)
SALAD:
    1/2 cup juice-packed peaches (50)
    1/4 cup strawberries, sliced (13)
    1 lettuce leaf (2)
Noncaloric beverage

### ALTERNATE
### DINNER MENU B: 490 CALORIES

* Southern Fried Chicken, Recipe #13 (255)
1 small potato (2 1/2-inch diameter,
    4 1/2 ounces), baked (90),
    topped with 2 tablespoons plain
    low-fat yogurt (19)
SALAD:
    1 cup chopped lettuce (9)
    3 slices tomato (21)
    1 tablespoon diet Italian dressing (6)
1 slice reduced-calorie bread (40)
1/2 cup unsweetened applesauce, heated (50),
    sprinkled with cinnamon
Noncaloric beverage

### ALTERNATE
### DINNER MENU C: 498 CALORIES

* Turkey Salad, Recipe #14 (188)
VEGETABLE PLATE:
    3 slices tomato (21)
    6 slices cucumber (4)
    6 carrot strips (12)
    drizzled with 1 tablespoon diet
    Italian dressing (6)
2 slices reduced-calorie bread (80)
*Peach Crumb Bake, Recipe #15 (97)
1 cup skim milk (90)

# =15=

# Recipes

Most of the recipes in the 32/32 diet require a minimum of preparation. You can shorten preparation time even more if you use a microwave instead of a  conventional oven. Either way, you'll find that the meals are nutritious, delicious, and filling.

The recipes are numbered consecutively to correspond with their appearance in the previous two chapters.

Recipe #1
BASIC BREAKFAST TWO

## TROPICAL BREAKFAST SHAKE

1/2 large banana (9³/4 inches long), frozen
3 ounces pineapple juice
1/2 cup skim milk
2 tablespoons wheat germ
1/2 teaspoon vanilla extract
1/2 teaspoon coconut flavoring
1 teaspoon vegetable oil
2 ice cubes (optional)

Peel banana, cut in half, wrap in aluminum foil, and freeze overnight. The next day, combine all ingredients, except ice cubes, in blender container or food processor. Cover; blend until smooth. If a thicker consistency is desired, add ice cubes and blend until thick and creamy. Serve immediately.

**Yield: 1 serving**
**Calories: 267**

Recipe #2

## MANDARIN CHICKEN

1/2 of a 9-ounce package frozen broccoli spears
1 whole chicken breast, boned, halved, and skinned
2 tablespoons flour
1/4 teaspoon garlic powder
1/8 teaspoon paprika
Butter-flavor cooking spray
1 1/2 tablespoons low-calorie margarine
1/2 cup orange juice
2 tablespoons sauterne cooking wine
1/2 teaspoon dried tarragon
1/2 teaspoon cornstarch
1/4 teaspoon grated orange peel
4.3-ounce can mandarin orange segments, drained

### Conventional oven:

Thaw broccoli in a bowl of warm water for 30 minutes; drain. Heat oven to 350 degrees. Flatten chicken breasts by pounding lightly between sheets of wax paper. Combine flour, garlic powder, and paprika in a small bowl. Coat chicken with flour mixture.

Treat a medium skillet with cooking spray, add margarine, and heat to melt. Brown chicken breasts over medium-high heat. Remove chicken and place in 8-inch (2-quart) square baking dish. Combine orange juice, cooking wine, tarragon, cornstarch, and orange peel in a container with a tight-fitting lid. Shake until blended; add to same skillet and cook until mixture boils and thickens, stirring constantly. Pour sauce over chicken.

Bake chicken at 350 degrees for 15 minutes. Divide broccoli into two equal portions; arrange on top of chicken breasts. Top each serving with mandarin oranges. Cover and bake an additional 15 minutes.

### Microwave:

Place broccoli in a small casserole with a lid, add 2 tablespoons of water and cook on high for 3 minutes; set aside. Flatten chicken breasts by pounding lightly between sheets of wax paper. Arrange chicken in an 8-inch (2-quart) square microwave-safe dish; sprinkle with garlic powder and paprika. Cover with waxed paper; microwave on HIGH for 4 minutes.

Combine orange juice, wine, tarragon, cornstarch, and orange peel in a 2-cup glass measuring cup or small bowl. Microwave on HIGH for 2 to 3 minutes or until thickened; pour over chicken. Divide broccoli into two equal portions; arrange on top of chicken breasts. Top each serving with mandarin oranges. Microwave on HIGH for 2 to 3 minutes or until chicken is thoroughly cooked.

**Yield: 2 servings**
**Calories: 315/serving**

Recipe #3

## VEGETABLE-TOPPED FISH FILLET

8 ounces fresh or individually frozen
   fish fillets
4 ounces tomato sauce
1/4 cup thinly sliced celery
1/4 cup chopped onion
1/4 cup sauterne cooking wine
1 clove garlic, minced
1/4 teaspoon salt
1/4 teaspoon dried basil, crushed
4 ounces snow pea pods (or English peas)
1/4 cup water
1 tablespoon cornstarch

Place fillets (do not thaw if frozen) in skillet. Combine tomato sauce, celery, onion, green pepper, wine, garlic, salt, and basil; add to skillet and bring to a boil. Reduce heat; cover and simmer 5 minutes or until fish is nearly done.

Meanwhile, divide the peas between two shallow individual baking dishes. Remove fish from skillet; place atop peas. Combine water and cornstarch in a container with a tight-fitting lid; shake until blended. Add mixture to skillet; cook and stir until bubbly. Spoon over fish. Continue cooking according to directions below or cover with foil and freeze.

### Conventional oven:
Bake, covered, at 375 degrees for 10 to 15 minutes. If reheating from frozen, bake covered at 375 degrees for 45 to 50 minutes or until hot.

### Microwave:
Cover with vented plastic wrap or waxed paper. Cook, covered, at MEDIUM-HIGH 2 to 3 minutes. If reheating from frozen, remove foil, cover with vented plastic wrap or waxed paper, and cook, covered, at MEDIUM-HIGH for 6 minutes, giving dish a half-turn once.

**Yield: 2 servings**
**Calories: 235/serving**

## Recipe #4

# WALDORF SPECIAL

1 small apple (unpeeled), chopped
1 tablespoon lemon juice
1 small pineapple, juice-packed, drained
    and chopped
1 tablespoon raisins
1 teaspoon low-calorie mayonnaise
1 lettuce leaf

Toss apple in lemon juice; drain. Add remaining ingredients, except lettuce, and mix lightly. Cover and chill. Serve on lettuce leaf.

**Yield: 1 serving**
**Calories: 129**

## Recipe #5

# CHEESY MACARONI

4 ounces uncooked macaroni
2 tablespoons flour
1 cup skim milk
2 ounces (3 slices) low-calorie cheddar
    cheese slices
Salt and pepper to taste

**Conventional oven:**
Cook macaroni to desired consistency as directed on package. Drain; rinse with hot water.

Combine flour and ½ cup skim milk in a container with a tight-fitting lid; shake until well blended. Pour into medium saucepan; add remaining milk. Cook over medium heat, stirring constantly until mixture boils and thickens. Add cheese; continue cooking until cheese is melted, stirring constantly. Add cooked macaroni, salt and pepper. Heat thoroughly.

**Microwave:**
Bring 3 cups of water to a boil (8 to 10 minutes on HIGH) in a 3-quart microwave-proof casserole. Add pasta to dish; cook 10 to 12 minutes on MEDIUM; drain and rinse with hot water.

Combine flour and 1/2 cup milk in deep microwave-proof bowl or 4-cup glass measure. Cook on HIGH for 1 minute or until warm; stir and repeat until thickening. Tear cheese into strips; stir into milk mixture until melted. Add remaining milk and macaroni, salt and pepper; cook on BAKE for 5 to 6 minutes or until mixture bubbles.

**Yield: 2 servings**
**Calories: 390/serving**

Recipe #6

# PEPPERS 'N' ONIONS

1 teaspoon reduced-calorie margarine
1 tablespoon low-sodium soy sauce
1/4 cup green peppers, chopped
1/4 cup onions, sliced

Melt margarine in a small skillet; stir in soy sauce. Add onions and peppers; cook until crisp-tender. Serve over steak.

**Yield: 1 serving**
**Calories: 40**

Recipe #7

# CHICKEN PEA BAKE

1/2 tablespoon reduced-calorie margarine,
 melted
1 teaspoon light soy sauce
3/4 teaspoon paprika
1/4 teaspoon dried poultry seasoning
1 whole chicken breast (about 8 ounces),
 divided and skinned
2 packages low-sodium chicken bouillon
1/4 cup sauterne cooking wine
1 1/2 cups hot water
1/4 pound fresh mushrooms, sliced
 and drained
4 ounces snow pea pods (or English peas),
 thawed and drained

## Conventional oven:

Combine first four ingredients in a shallow 2-quart casserole. Place chicken in casserole, turning to coat.

Mix bouillon, wine, and water in a small bowl. Add mushrooms to casserole; pour bouillon around chicken. Cover and bake at 350 degrees for 50 minutes. Add peas; cover and bake an additional 10 minutes or until peas are tender.

## Microwave:

Place margarine in a 2-quart microwave-proof casserole and heat on HIGH for 15 to 20 seconds or until melted; add next three ingredients. Place chicken in casserole, turning to coat.

Mix water, wine, and bouillon in a small bowl. Add mushrooms to casserole; pour bouillon around chicken. Cover and cook breast-side down on HIGH 3 to 4 minutes. Turn chicken over; add peas; cover and cook on HIGH 3 to 4 minutes. Let stand 5 minutes.

**Yield: 2 servings**
**Calories: 216/serving**

Recipe #8

# APPLE CHOPS

2 lean center-cut pork chops, fat trimmed
　　(about 1/2-inch thick)
1/8 teaspoon garlic powder
1/8 teaspoon pepper
Butter-flavor cooking spray
1/2 cup unsweetened apple juice
1 tablespoon grated onion
1 medium-sweet red apple (3-inch diameter),
　　cored, sliced
1 tablespoon flour

## Conventional stove:

Sprinkle chops with garlic powder and pepper. Treat large skillet with cooking spray; brown chops on both sides over medium heat. Add 1/4 cup apple juice and onion to chops. Cover; simmer 50 to 60 minutes or until tender. Remove chops; cover and keep warm. Stir flour into reserved apple juice until smooth. Bring liquid in skillet to a boil; stir in flour mixture. Cook over low heat, stirring constantly until thickened. Stir in apples; cook until thoroughly heated. Serve over chops.

## Microwave:

Brown chops as instructed above. Transfer to a large microwave-proof casserole; add 1/4 cup apple juice and onion to chops. Cover; cook on HIGH 5 to 7 minutes. Remove chops; cover and keep warm. Stir flour into reserved apple juice until smooth; add to casserole and cook on HIGH for 1 minute. Stir and repeat until thickened; add apples. Heat on HIGH for 1 minute until thoroughly heated. Serve over chops.

**Yield: 2 servings**
**Calories: 254/serving**

Recipe #9

## QUICK & EASY LASAGNA

(Note: recipe yields 8 servings)

32 ounces Italian sauce (see recipe on next page)
1 cup water (3/4 cup for microwave cooking)
16-ounce carton low-fat cottage cheese
2 tablespoons chopped chives (fresh or dried)
1 egg
8 ounces uncooked lasagna noodles
12-ounce package part-skim mozzarella cheese
2 tablespoons grated Parmesan cheese

**Conventional oven:**
Add Italian sauce to water; blend well. Simmer 5 minutes. While sauce is heating, beat cottage cheese with hand mixer until smooth. Combine cottage cheese, chives, and egg in a medium bowl. Spread 1 1/2 cups of sauce in the bottom of a 13-inch by 9-inch (3-quart) baking dish or lasagna pan. Top with 1/2 of noodles, 1/2 of cheese mixture and 1/2 of mozzarella cheese. Repeat layers. Top with remaining sauce; sprinkle with Parmesan.

Cover with aluminum foil and bake at 350 degrees for 50 to 55 minutes. Remove foil and continue baking for an additional 5 minutes or until casserole is bubbly. Let stand 15 minutes before serving.

**Microwave:**
Assemble casserole as directed above in a microwave-proof 3-quart casserole. Cover with vented plastic or wax paper; cook on HIGH for 20 minutes, turning a quarter-turn after every 5 minutes. Let stand 15 minutes before serving.

**Yield: 8 servings**
**Calories: 356/serving**

## ITALIAN SAUCE

24 ounces canned tomato sauce
20 ounces canned stewed tomatoes
Medium onion, chopped
1/2 pound fresh mushrooms, sliced
1/2 teaspoon dried Italian seasoning
Dash garlic powder
Salt and pepper to taste

Combine all ingredients in a heavy saucepan; simmer, uncovered, 45 minutes. (Divide leftovers into individual 1/2-cup serving-size freezer containers; freeze. Thaw and use when needed.)

**Yield: approximately 5 cups**
**Calories: 35/one-half cup**
(already counted into Lasagna recipe)

Recipe #10

## SWEET 'N' SOUR MEATBALLS

5 ounces lean ground beef
4 saltines, crushed
1/4 teaspoon salt
1/8 teaspoon ginger
Dash pepper
1 egg, slightly beaten
8 ounces pineapple chunks, juice-packed,
    drained, reserving liquid
2 tablespoons brown sugar substitute
1 1/2 tablespoons cider vinegar
1 tablespoon low-sodium soy sauce
1/2 cup diagonally sliced carrots
1/2 medium green pepper, sliced
1/2 tablespoon cornstarch
2 tablespoons water

**Conventional stove:**
Combine ground beef, cracker crumbs, salt, ginger, pepper, and egg; form into 1-inch balls. Place meatballs in large skillet and brown, turning fre-

quently; drain. Add enough water to reserved pineapple liquid to equal $1/2$ cup, then add brown sugar, cider vinegar, and soy sauce, and blend well. Pour sauce over meatballs; stir in carrots. Bring to a boil. Reduce heat; cover and simmer 10 to 15 minutes or until carrots are crisp-tender. Stir in green pepper and pineapple; cover and simmer 5 minutes. Combine cornstarch and water in a small bowl; gradually add to skillet, stirring constantly until thickened. Serve over hot cooked rice.

**Microwave:**

Prepare meatballs as directed above. Place meatballs in a single layer in an oblong microwave-proof baking dish. Cook, uncovered, on BAKE for 4 minutes, turning frequently; drain. Add enough water to reserved pineapple liquid to equal $1/2$ cup, then add brown sugar substitute, cider vinegar, and soy sauce, and blend well. Pour sauce over meatballs; mix in carrots, green pepper, and pineapple. Cover and cook 3 to 5 minutes on HIGH. Combine cornstarch and water in a small bowl; blend well. Stir into meatballs. Cover and cook on SIMMER 4 to 6 minutes or until vegetables are tender and sauce is thickened. Let stand 3 minutes. Serve over hot cooked rice.

**Yield: 2 servings**
**Calories: 298/serving**

## Recipe #11

# HUEVOS RANCHEROS

1 6-inch corn tortilla
$1/2$ of a 10-ounce can tomatoes and
    green chili peppers
1 egg, large
1 egg white
$1/2$ ounce shredded Monterey Jack cheese
$1/2$ ounce part-skim mozzarella cheese
2 tablespoons plain low-fat yogurt
$1/2$ tablespoon chives

Brush tortilla lightly with water to make it more pliable. Press tortilla into a small individual casserole. Bake at 350 degrees for 15 minutes or until tortilla is crisp.

Meanwhile, bring tomatoes and chilis to a boil; reduce heat. Beat egg and egg white lightly; carefully pour into the skillet. Cover and cook over low heat about 5 minutes or to desired doneness.

Carefully slide the egg and tomato mixture into the warm tortilla. Sprinkle with cheese; return to oven about 1 minute more or until cheese melts.

Remove from oven. Top with yogurt and sprinkle with chives.

**Yield: 1 serving**
**Calories: 272**

## Recipe #12

# SPANISH RICE

Butter-flavor cooking spray
1/2 tablespoon vegetable oil
2 tablespoons onion, chopped
1/8 teaspoon garlic powder
Salt to taste
1/2 of a 10-ounce can tomatoes and
　　green chili peppers
2 packages chicken bouillon
1/8 teaspoon chili powder
1 cup water
1/2 cup uncooked rice

### Conventional stove:
Treat medium saucepan with cooking spray; add oil, onion, garlic powder, and salt. Cook and stir until onion is tender. Add tomatoes and green chilis, chicken bouillon, chili powder, and water; blend well. Bring mixture to a boil; stir in rice. Cover and let stand over very low heat 15 to 20 minutes or until liquid is absorbed.

### Microwave:
Treat 2-quart microwave-proof casserole with cooking spray; add oil, onion, garlic powder, and salt. Cook 1 minute on HIGH. Add remaining ingredients, except rice; cover and cook on HIGH for 5 minutes or until boiling. Stir in rice; cover and cook on SIMMER for 10 to 15 minutes or until liquid is absorbed. Let stand, covered, for 5 minutes.

**Yield: 2 servings**
**Calories: 159/serving**

Recipe #13

# SOUTHERN FRIED CHICKEN

2 tablespoons low-calorie margarine,
   melted
1/4 cup (1 ounce) cornflake crumbs
1/2 tablespoon chopped chives
1/2 tablespoon chopped parsley
1 whole chicken breast (about 8 ounces),
   divided and skinned

### Conventional oven:

Place melted margarine in an 8-inch square baking dish. Combine corn-flake crumbs, chives, and parsley in a shallow dish. Dip chicken in margarine and roll in crumb mixture. Return chicken to baking dish, rib side up, and bake at 350 degrees for 30 minutes. Turn chicken and bake on the other side for 30 minutes.

### Microwave:

Place margarine in an 8-inch square microwave-proof baking dish. Cook on ROAST for 1 1/2 minutes or until margarine is melted. Combine cornflake crumbs, chives, and parsley in a shallow dish. Dip chicken in margarine and roll in crumb mixture. Return chicken to baking dish, breast side up, with the thickest side toward the outside of dish. Cover with waxed paper and cook on HIGH for 15 to 17 minutes or until chicken is tender. Let stand, covered, about 5 minutes before serving.

**Yield: 2 servings**
**Calories: 255/serving**

Recipe #14

# TURKEY SALAD

1 can (5 ounces) chunk white turkey, drained
3/4 cup unpeeled apple, chopped
1/2 cup celery, sliced
2 tablespoons raisins
1/3 cup diet Italian dressing
1 tablespoon brown sugar substitute

Gently stir together turkey, apple, celery, and raisins in a medium bowl. Mix dressing and brown sugar substitute in a measuring cup. Toss gently to coat. Serve on lettuce leaves.

**Yield: 2 servings**
**Calories: 188/serving**

Recipe #15

# PEACH CRUMB BAKE

> 1/2 cup peaches, juice-packed
> 1/2 graham cracker (2 sections), crushed
> Dash cinnamon
> Dash nutmeg
> 1 teaspoon low-calorie margarine, melted

Heat oven to 350 degrees. Place peaches in bottom of an 8-ounce custard cup. Combine graham cracker crumbs, cinnamon, and nutmeg in a small dish; mix well. Blend in margarine. Sprinkle mixture over peaches. Bake, uncovered, for 20 minutes. Serve warm.

**Yield: 1 serving**
**Calories: 97**

# =16=
# Shopping List

The following shopping list contains everything one person needs to follow the 32/32 menus and recipes for Days 1-16.

Staples, packaged goods, and frozen foods will last for many weeks and, if you prefer, can be purchased in quantities greater than those listed on an eight-day basis. Some produce should not be bought more than a week in advance. Poultry, meat, and especially fish will remain fresh for only a few days unless you freeze them.

When you bring the groceries home, keep perishability in mind and freeze certain items if necessary. Check your supplies at the end of each eight days.

Quantities needed for items marked with an asterisk (*) will depend on your individual selections for Basic Breakfasts and Basic Lunches. Review your choices and adjust the shopping list accordingly. You can modify these selections every eight days.

## DAYS 1-16

### STAPLES

* Noncaloric beverages (water, coffee, tea, diet soft drinks)
* Low-sodium bouillon, beef
* Low-sodium bouillon, chicken
Reduced-calorie bread (40 calories/slice)
* Cereal (110 calories per ounce), choose from:
Nabisco Shredded Wheat
Kellogg's Frosted Mini Wheats
Kellogg's NutriGrain Wheat or Corn
Post Grape Nuts

Ralston Purina Almond Delight
Ralston Purina Sun Flakes Crispy Wheat & Rice
Oatmeal
Quaker Oat Bran
Mozzarella cheese, part-skim, 16 ounces
Parmesan cheese
Graham crackers
Low-calorie margarine (50 calories per tablespoon)
Low-calorie mayonnaise (40 calories per tablespoon)
* Pineapple juice
Raisins
* Saltines
Skim milk
Vegetable cooking oil
Vegetable cooking spray (butter flavor)
* Wheat germ
Peanut butter
* Vanilla extract
* Coconut flavoring

## FRUITS, VEGETABLES, JUICES

Apple juice, unsweetened, 1 cup
* Red apple, medium (3-inch diameter)
Apples, 2 small (2$\frac{1}{2}$-inch diameter)
* Applesauce, unsweetened
Banana, 3 medium (8$\frac{3}{4}$ inches long)
* Banana, large (9$\frac{3}{4}$ inches long)
* Blueberries, fresh or frozen ($\frac{2}{3}$-cup serving)
Broccoli spears, frozen, 9-ounce package
Broccoli, chopped, 1 cup (fresh or frozen)
* Cantaloupe, fresh or frozen ($\frac{2}{3}$-cup serving)
Carrots
Celery
Green beans, French-style, fresh or frozen, 1$\frac{3}{4}$ cups
Corn, 1 ear (5 inches long)
Green pepper, 1 medium
* Lettuce, 1 large head
Mandarin oranges, canned, 4.3 ounces

Mushrooms, fresh, 1 pound
Onion, white, 2 medium (3-inch diameter)
Orange juice, unsweetened, 1/2 cup
Peach, medium (6 ounces, 2 3/4-inch diameter) or
　juice-packed peaches
Canned pineapple, juice-packed, 6 slices
Potatoes, 2 small (2 1/2-inch diameter, 4 1/2 ounces)
Sweet potato (5 inches long, 2-inch diameter)
Snow peas (or English peas), fresh or frozen, 8 ounces
Spinach, fresh leaves, 1 cup
* Strawberries (fresh or frozen without sugar), 1/2 cup
Canned stewed tomatoes, 20 ounces
Canned tomato sauce, 36 ounces
Tomatoes, 5 medium (3-inch diameter)
Pineapple chunks, juice-packed, 8 ounces

### BREADS, CEREALS

White rice, 1/4 cup uncooked
Lasagna noodles, 8 ounces dry
Macaroni, 4 ounces dry

### HERBS, SPICES, SEASONINGS

Dried basil
Chives (fresh or dried)
Cinnamon
Garlic cloves, 2
Garlic powder
Ginger
Grated orange peel
Dried Italian seasoning
Lemon juice
Paprika
Dried parsley
Dried poultry seasoning
Dried thyme
Dried tarragon

## MEAT, FISH, POULTRY

Whole chicken breasts, 2 ( raw weight 8 ounces each)
Eggs, 2 large
Fish fillet, fresh or frozen, 8 ounces
Lean ground beef, 5 ounces
Lean sirloin, 3 ounces
  * Lean roast beef, sliced (2-ounce serving)
  * Turkey, roasted, skinned (2-ounce serving)
  * Tuna, water-packed (6¹/2-ounce can)
Lean center-cut pork chops, fat trimmed, 2 (¹/2-inch thick)

## DAIRY PRODUCTS

  * Low-fat American cheese (1¹/2 slices = 50 calories), 1 ounce
  * Low-fat cheddar cheese (1¹/2 slices = 50 calories), 3 slices
Low-fat cottage cheese, 16 ounces
Low-fat vanilla yogurt
Low-fat plain yogurt

## MISCELLANEOUS

Brown sugar substitute
Cornstarch
Diet Italian dressing (6 calories per tablespoon)
Low-sodium soy sauce
Sauterne cooking wine, 5 ounces
  * Light beer (95 calories), no more than 3 for 8 days
Popcorn (plain or packaged for microwave), 2 cups popped
Flour
Cider vinegar

For Days 17-32, the preceding shopping list applies. In addition, you might wish to purchase the following items.

# SHOPPING LIST FOR ALTERNATE DINNER MENUS

## FRUITS, VEGETABLES, JUICES

Apple, 1
Applesauce, unsweetened, 1/2 cup
Canned peaches, juice-packed, 1/2 cup
Canned tomatoes and green chilies, 10-ounce can
Lettuce
Onion, chopped
Potato (21/2-inch diameter, 41/2 ounces)
Raisins, 2 tablespoons
Strawberries
Tomato, 1 medium

## BREADS, CEREALS

Corn tortilla (6 inch), 1
Cornflakes, 1 ounce
White rice, uncooked, 1/2 cup
Graham cracker, 1/2 (2 sections)
Reduced-calorie bread, 3 slices

## HERBS, SPICES, SEASONINGS

Chives
Chili powder
Parsley
Nutmeg

## MEAT, FISH, POULTRY

Eggs, 2 large
Chicken breast, whole (about 8 ounces)
Canned chunk white turkey, 5 ounces

## DAIRY PRODUCTS

Monterey Jack cheese, 1/2 ounce
Mozzarella cheese, part-skim, 1/2 ounce
Low-fat plain yogurt, 8 ounces
Skim milk, 1 cup

# =17=
# Troubleshooting

It is no secret that some men hate to shop and cook. I feel strongly that if you fall into this category, you should *do it anyway*—at least for the first eight days. Even if your spouse or someone else usually shops and cooks for you, you need to visit the supermarket with her, start reading the nutrition information labels on packaged foods, and become involved in the weighing, measuring, preparing, and cooking of the recommended menus. The experience will demonstrate the importance of serving sizes and calories. If your cooking tolerance remains low, the rest of this troubleshooting chapter will help you.

## LEAN CUISINE
## RECOMMENDATIONS

The following Lean Cuisine frozen dinners may be substituted for any of the 500-calorie evening meals.

- Lean Cuisine Chicken with Vegetables (270)
  2 slices low-calorie bread (80)
  2 teaspoons low-calorie margarine (34)
  1 cup skim milk (90)

- Lean Cuisine Zucchini Lasagna (260)
  2 slices low-calorie bread (80)
  2 teaspoons low-calorie margarine (34)
  1 cup skim milk (90)

- Lean Cuisine Filet of Fish Divan (260)
  2 slices low-calorie bread (80)
  2 teaspoons low-calorie margarine (34)
  1 cup skim milk (90)

# OTHER ACCEPTABLE
# ENTREES

Other frozen dinners that may be used in place of the 32/32 dinner menus are as follows:

### Weight Watchers
    Chicken Ala King
    Imperial Chicken and Mushrooms
    Pasta Rigati in Meat Sauce
    Sweet 'n Sour Chicken Tenders

### Mrs. Paul's Light Entrees
    Shrimp Primavera
    Tuna Pasta Casserole

### Budget Gourmet's
    Mandarin Chicken

### Benihana's
    Chicken in Spicy Garlic Sauce

These frozen entrees, when consumed with 2 slices of low-calorie bread, 2 teaspoons of low-calorie margarine, and 1 cup of skim milk, have the proper proportions of carbohydrates, fats, and proteins. Even so, you should use the frozen entrees no more than four times per week.

# FAST FOOD
# FOR TRAVELERS

Two other  substitutions were useful to the 32/32 dieters in Dallas, especially those who were frequent travelers. The following fast foods may be used in place of a 500-calorie evening meal:

- Two McDonald's small hamburgers, all but one bite (526)
  Diet coke (1)

- Burger King's Whopper Jr. (322)
  1 cup whole milk (150)

As with the frozen entrees, you should substitute the hamburgers no more than four times per week.

## ACT PRUDENTLY

The key to success with food substitutions is to employ them prudently. Use them to your advantage, and your fat-loss results will accelerate.

# _=18=_
# 32/32 Nautilus Routines

Nautilus machines are large, heavy-duty exercise devices made of tubular steel by Nautilus Sports/Medical Industries, Inc. They come in various shapes, sizes, and colors, and there are separate machines for each major muscle group. Behind Nautilus is scientific thinking that makes Nautilus exercise safer and more efficient at building muscle than traditional forms of lifting with barbells and dumbbells.

If you have access to Nautilus equipment, you'll get better results.

Most of the 146 men I supervised through the 32/32 program in Dallas, Texas, exercised on Nautilus equipment. Each man added an average of 3.65 pounds of muscle to his physique in just 32 days. Such gains not only made each man look better, but increased his metabolic rate by approximately 275 calories per day. Remember, building your muscles is a major factor in keeping your lost fat off permanently.

The super-slow Nautilus program centers around three nonconsecutive-day, 20-minute workouts per week. You perform only eight exercises during Days 1-16. Days 17-32 require a maximum of ten exercises.

With the workouts, you'll be amazed at how much stronger you become in only 32 days. If you also adhere to the diet, you'll be elated by your fat loss and the tightness and muscularity beginning to show throughout your midsection.

As was noted in Chapter 7, when you can perform eight or more super-slow repetitions on any exercise, you should increase the weight by 5 percent at your next workout. Strive to make progress at each successive workout.

## TESTING
## YOUR STRENGTH

I recommend testing your starting level of strength on four Nautilus machines: leg extension and leg curl for your lower body, pullover and abdominal for your upper body.

Through trial and error during the first two workouts, determine the maximum weight you can lift for six super-slow repetitions on the above four machines. Add the weight on the leg extension to the weight on the leg curl and divide by two. This is your starting lower body strength.

Add the weight used on the pullover to the weight used on the abdominal and divide by two to calculate your upper body strength.

Repeat this procedure when the 32-day program is over. Expect an increase in strength of 30 to 40 percent in both your upper and lower body.

## WARMING UP AND
## COOLING DOWN

Before exercising on Nautilus equipment, or with free weights, take several minutes to warm up. Do some light calisthenics or ride a stationary bicycle for five minutes. After your workout, cool down by walking around the exercise area, getting a drink of water, and moving your arms in slow circles. Continue these easy movements for three to four minutes until your heart rate subsides.

## THE BEST NAUTILUS
## ROUTINES

The following routines were used by the men in Dallas with outstanding results. If certain machines are not at your disposal, substitutions can be made. For example, you can substitute the Duo Hip and Back for the Lower Back, the Decline Press for the Bench Press, or the Duo Leg Press for the Calf Raise. Be sure to check with your local Nautilus instructor for assistance in using any unfamiliar Nautilus machines.

Following are the recommended Nautilus routines.

| **DAYS 1-16** | **DAYS 17-32** |
|---|---|

1. Leg Curl
2. Leg Extension
3. Lateral Raise
4. Pullover
5. Multi-Biceps
6. Abdominal
7. Lower Back
8. Rotary Torso

1. Leg Curl
2. Leg Extension
3. Calf Raise on Multi-Exercise*
4. Lateral Raise
5. Bench Press*
6. Pullover
7. Multi-Biceps
8. Abdominal
9. Lower Back
10. Rotary Torso

*Indicates new exercise

## LEG CURL

### contracted position

LEG CURL for back thighs: Lie face down on the machine. Place your feet under the roller pads and your knees barely over the edge of the bench. Grasp the handles to stabilize your body. Curl both legs slowly upward in 10 seconds. Try to touch your buttocks with the roller pads. Pause in the contracted position. Lower the resistance in 5 seconds. Repeat for maximum repetitions.

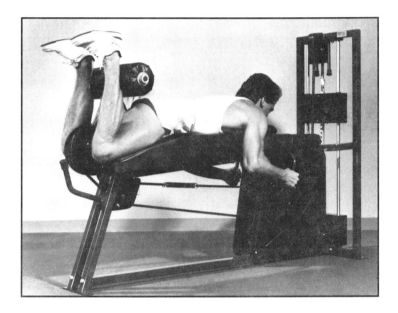

## LEG EXTENSION

### contracted position

L̲E̲G̲ ̲E̲X̲T̲E̲N̲S̲I̲O̲N̲ for front thighs: Sit in the machine. Place your ankles behind the roller pads, with your knees snug against the seat bottom and your torso against the seat back. Some shorter men may require a long pad to be positioned between their buttocks and the seat back. Fasten the seat belt across your hips. Grasp the handles lightly. Straighten both legs slowly in 10 seconds. Pause. Lower your legs in 5 seconds. Repeat for maximum repetitions.

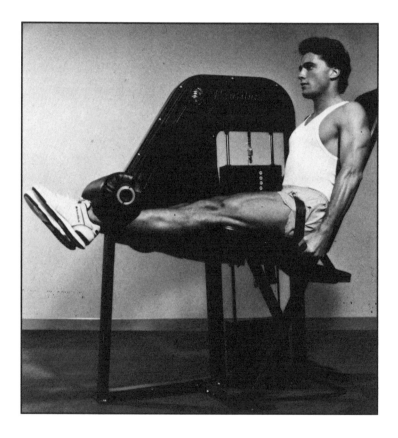

## CALF RAISE ON MULTI-EXERCISE

### contracted position

CALF RAISE for back calves: Attach the steel ring of the padded belt to the hook snap on the movement arm of the multi-exercise machine. Grasping the padded belt, place both feet through the middle while facing the machine, and kneel on the first step. Position the belt around your hips and stand up smoothly. Place the balls of your feet on the first step and your hands on the front of the carriage. Lock your knees and keep them locked throughout the movement. Elevate your heels as high as possible in 10 seconds and try to stand on your tiptoes. Lower your heels in 5 seconds and stretch. Repeat for maximum repetitions.

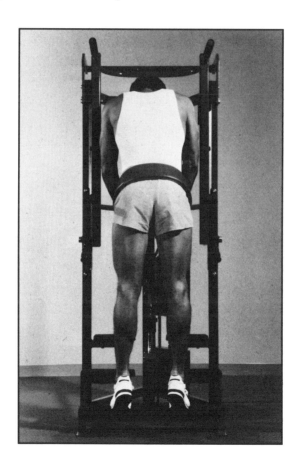

## LATERAL RAISE

### contracted position

LATERAL RAISE for shoulders: Adjust the seat until your shoulder joints are in line with the axes of rotation of the movement arms. Fasten the seat belt. Pull your knees together and cross your ankles. Position your elbows slightly to the rear of your torso, inside the movement arm pads. Grasp the handles lightly. Pressing against the movement arm pads, raise your elbows slowly to ear level in 10 seconds. Pause briefly in the top position. Lower your elbows to your sides in 5 seconds. Repeat for maximum repetitions.

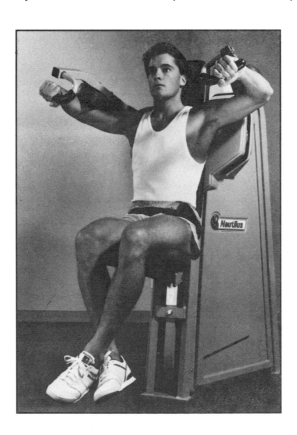

## BENCH PRESS

**top position**

B̲E̲N̲C̲H̲ ̲P̲R̲E̲S̲S̲ for chest, shoulders, and upper arms: Lie face up on the bench with the handles beside your chest. Grasp the handles lightly. Stabilize your body by placing your feet flat on the floor, or on the step at the end of the bench. Press the handles upward slowly in 10 seconds. Lower the handles in 5 seconds. Repeat for maximum repetitions.

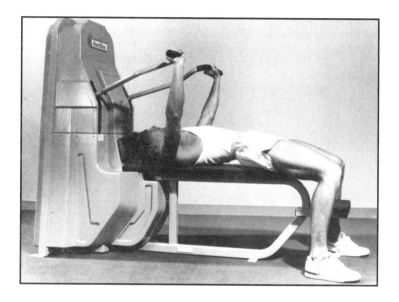

## PULLOVER

### stretched position

PULLOVER for upper back: Adjust the seat so your shoulders are in line with the axes of rotation of the movement arm. Assume an erect position and fasten the seat belt. Leg press the foot pedal until the elbow pads approach chin level. Place your elbows on the pads and your hands against the curved portion of the crossbar. Remove your feet from the pedal and rotate your elbows back for a comfortable stretch. This is the starting position. Rotate your shoulders forward and down in 10 seconds. Pause with the bar touching your midsection. Return to the stretched position in 5 seconds. Repeat for maximum repetitions.

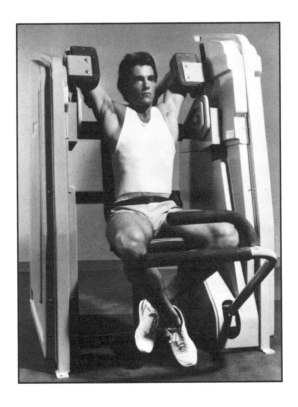

## MULTI-BICEPS

### midrange position

MULTI-BICEPS for upper arms: Stand and place your elbows on the horizontal pad in line with the axes of the movement arms. Grasp the handles lightly. Bend your arms to 90 degrees and be seated. Lower the handles until your arms are straight. Your elbows should be slightly higher than your shoulders. If not, relax your arms and readjust the seat. Curl both handles slowly in 10 seconds. Your thumbs should almost touch your shoulders. Pause. Lower the handles to the stretched position in 5 seconds. Repeat for maximum repetitions.

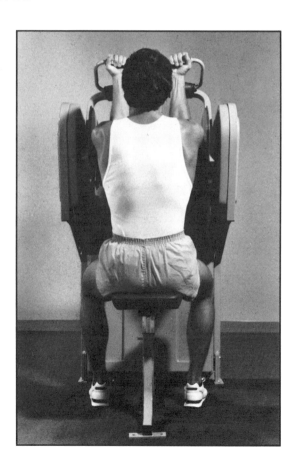

## ABDOMINAL

### contracted position

ABDOMINAL for front waist: Adjust the seat until your navel is approximately parallel to the center of the raised Nautilus shell on the side of the plastic shield. Fasten the seat belt across your hips. Pull your knees together and cross your ankles. Place your elbows on the pads and lightly grasp the handles. Expand your chest, pull gradually with your elbows, and slowly shorten the distance between your rib cage and pelvis in 10 seconds. Pause in the contracted position. Return to the starting position in 5 seconds. Repeat for maximum repetitions.

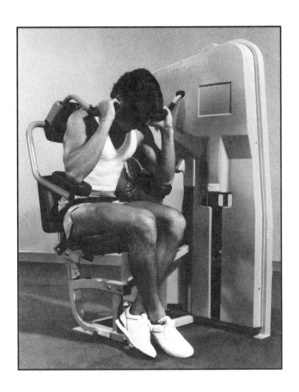

## LOWER BACK
### contracted position

Lower back for lower back: Sit in the machine with your buttocks as far back in the seat as possible. Adjust the foot board so your knees are slightly bent and place your feet on the platform. During the movement you must keep your buttocks stationary against the seat by pushing back with your feet and thighs; your knees must remain slightly bent to do this properly. Fasten the seat belt snugly across your hips. Position your middle back against the pad on its movement arm. Interlace your fingers across your waist. Move your torso slowly backward in 10 seconds. The range of movement is short. Pause in the contracted position. Return to the starting position in 5 seconds. Repeat for maximum repetitions.

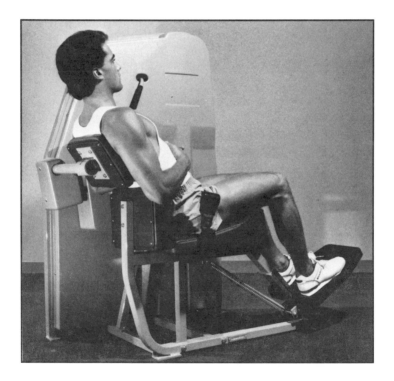

## ROTARY TORSO

### contracted position

ROTARY TORSO for sides of waist: Position your head and spine directly above the pivot point of the movement arm. Straddle the seat. Anchor your lower body by crossing your ankles and squeezing the pad between your knees. Fasten the belt securely across your thighs. Place your upper arms securely over the angled roller pads behind your back. Your elbows should be as close together as comfortably possible. Rotate your torso from the starting position to the opposite side in 10 seconds. Pause. Return to the starting position in 5 seconds. Repeat for maximum repetitions. After completing this part of the exercise, unlock the seat and move it to the opposite side of the machine. Go through the same procedure for the other side.

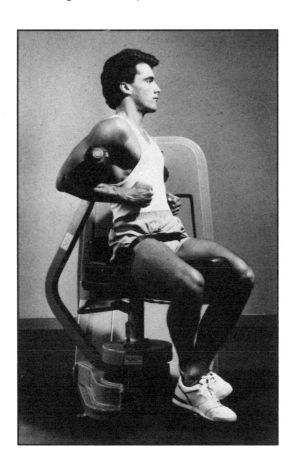

# _=19=_
# 32/32 Free-Weight Routines

If it is inconvenient for you to train on Nautilus equipment, and you don't already have a barbell set in the garage, you should locate a free-weight facility. You can get very adequate muscle-building results from free weights. Small groups of men who completed the 32/32 program using free weights instead of Nautilus produced approximately 80 percent of the muscle-building gains of similar Nautilus groups.

The key to getting results is not so much in the equipment—but in *how you use it*.

The best way to use Nautilus, free weights, and most other resistance equipment, is with a super-slow, high-intensity style.

For the 32/32 free-weight routines, you'll need an adjustable barbell and dumbbell and weight plates in increments of 1 1/4, 2 1/2, 5, 10, and 25 pounds. A bench and squat rack are valuable accessories for anyone serious about training.

Use resistance on the recommended exercises that permits you to perform one set of four to eight super-slow repetitions. When you can accomplish eight or more repetitions in proper form, increase the weight by 5 percent at the time of your next workout. Each workout should be intense, brief, and repeated approximately three times per week.

Following are the suggested free-weight routines.

| **DAYS 1-16** | **DAYS 17-32** |
|---|---|
| 1. Squat with barbell | 1. Squat with barbell |
| 2. Pullover with dumbbell | 2. Pullover with dumbbell |
| 3. Calf raise on one leg with dumbbell | 3. Calf raise on one leg with dumbbell |
| 4. Shoulder shrug with barbell | 4. Shoulder shrug with barbell |
| 5. Overhead press with barbell | 5. Overhead press with barbell |
| 6. Biceps curl with barbell | 6. Bent-over rowing with barbell* |
| 7. Trunk curl | 7. Bench press with barbell* |
| 8. Side bend with dumbbell | 8. Biceps curl |
| | 9. Trunk curl |
| | 10. Side bend with dumbbell |

* Indicates new exercise

## SQUAT WITH BARBELL

**bottom position**

SQUAT for hips, lower back, and thighs: Stand erect, feet shoulder-width apart, with a barbell secured in your hands and balanced across your shoulders. Some men may need a 2-by-6-inch board to elevate their heels for better balance. Lower your upper body in 5 seconds by bending your knees and hips. Look straight ahead and keep your back flat during the movement. Continue downward until your thighs come in contact with the backs of your calves. Do not relax or bounce at the bottom. Return to an almost-erect position very slowly in 10 seconds. Keep your knees slightly bent at the top. This makes the exercise more demanding. Repeat for maximum repetitions.

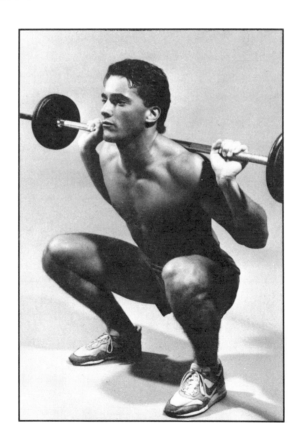

## PULLOVER WITH DUMBBELL

### starting position

PULLOVER for upper back: Lie across a sturdy bench with your back in the middle and your head and hips off the sides. With both hands, hold one end of a dumbbell over your chest with your arms straight. Lower the dumbbell over your head toward the floor. Do not bend elbows. Stretch in the bottom position. Lift the dumbbell back over your chest slowly in 10 seconds. Repeat for maximum repetitions.

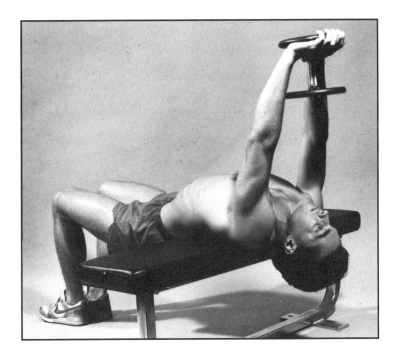

## CALF RAISE ON
## ONE LEG WITH DUMBBELL

### contracted position

CALF RAISE ON ONE LEG for back calf: Position ball of your left foot on the edge of several stacked weight plates, or on a 2-by-6 board placed flat on the floor. Lock your left knee and suspend your other foot. Steady your balance by holding onto the back of a chair with your left hand. Hold a light dumbbell in your right hand. Raise your left heel slowly in 10 seconds and stand on your tiptoes. Lower smoothly to a deep stretch in 5 seconds. Repeat for maximum repetitions. Follow the same procedure for your right calf.

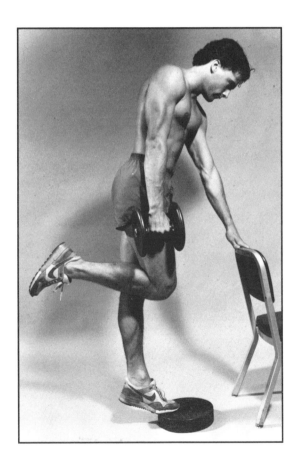

## SHOULDER SHRUG WITH BARBELL

**contracted position**

SHOULDER SHRUG for middle and upper back: Grasp a barbell with an overhand grip and stand. Keeping your arms straight, slowly shrug your shoulders in 10 seconds as high as possible. Pause in the top position. Lower smoothly in 5 seconds. Repeat for maximum repetitions.

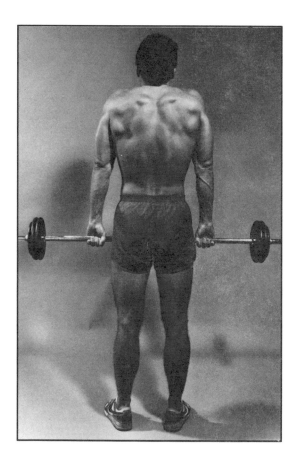

## OVERHEAD PRESS WITH BARBELL

**starting position**

OVERHEAD PRESS for shoulders: Lift the barbell to your shoulders. Your hands should be shoulder-width apart. Press the barbell overhead in 10 seconds. Lower back to your shoulders in 5 seconds. Repeat for maximum repetitions.

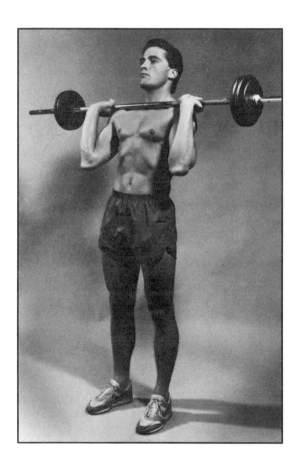

## BENT-OVER ROWING WITH BARBELL

**contracted position**

B̲E̲N̲T̲-O̲V̲E̲R̲ ̲R̲O̲W̲I̲N̲G̲ for back: From a standing position, bend over and grasp a barbell with a narrow grip. Your torso should be parallel to the floor. Pull the barbell upward in 10 seconds until it touches your midsection. Pause. Lower to the starting position in 5 seconds. Repeat for maximum repetitions.

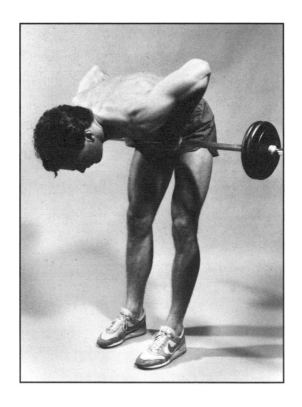

## BENCH PRESS WITH BARBELL

### midrange position

Bench press for chest, shoulders, and upper arms: A bench with an attached barbell rack produces the best results. Lie face up on the bench and position your shoulders under the barbell. Adjust your hands on the barbell until they are slightly wider than your shoulders. Lift the barbell from the rack and bring it over your chest. Lower the barbell to your chest in 5 seconds. Press it slowly back to the starting position in 10 seconds. Repeat for maximum repetitions.

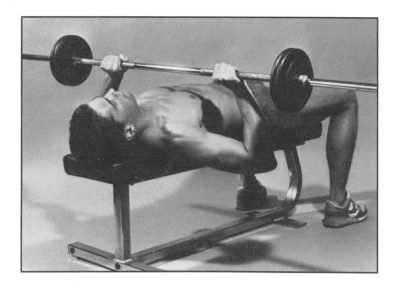

## BICEPS CURL WITH BARBELL
### midrange position

BICEPS CURL for upper arms: Grasp a barbell with an underhand grip and stand. Stabilize your elbows by your sides. Curl barbell slowly to shoulder height in 10 seconds. Lower to starting position in 5 seconds. Repeat for maximum repetitions.

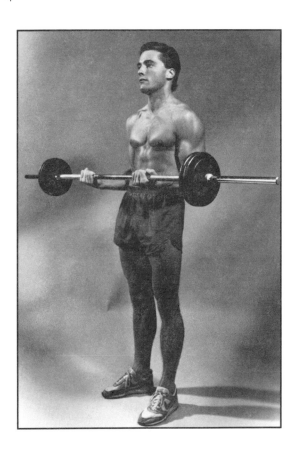

## TRUNK CURL

### contracted position

Trunk curl for midsection: Lie face up on the floor with your hands behind your head. Bring your heels close to your buttocks and spread your knees. Try lifting your shoulders and back off the floor as far as possible and hold the top position for 10 seconds. Lower your shoulders back to the floor in 5 seconds. Repeat for maximum repetitions.

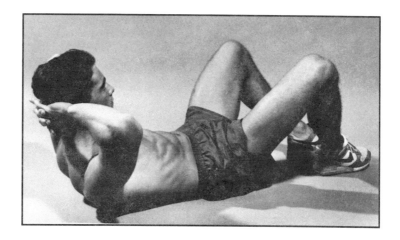

## SIDE BEND WITH DUMBBELL

### stretched position

SIDE BEND for sides of waist: Grasp a dumbbell in your right hand and stand erect. Place your left hand on your head. Bend to your right side as far as possible in 5 seconds. Lift the dumbbell slowly back to the standing position in 10 seconds. Repeat for maximum repetitions. Change the dumbbell to your left hand and work the other side.

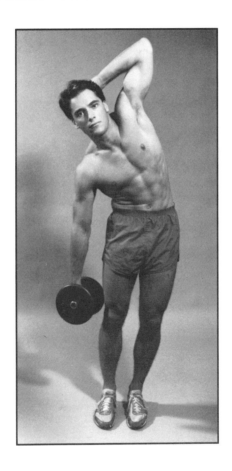

# —=20=—

# 32 Little Ways to Lose Those Last 5 Pounds

Those last few pounds, those last few fractions of an inch around your waist, always seem the hardest to lose. Here are 32 little ways to reach your goal more efficiently. These hints will also help you in long-term maintenance.

1. Go grocery shopping only on a full stomach.

2. Shop from a written list of necessities. Walking through the supermarket unprepared can be hazardous to your health.

3. Pace your eating by putting your fork down between bites. The more slowly you eat, the more quickly you'll feel full.

4. Use whipped or softened butter or margarine. You'll get the same flavor for less fat.

5. Learn to say "No, thank you" when people offer you food.

6. Hold a conference and explain your fat-loss program to family, friends, and co-workers.

7. Drink no-calorie sparkling waters when you're out, instead of alcoholic beverages.

8. Set realistic goals, then take them one day at a time.

9. Don't use place settings with intense colors such as warm red, bright yellow, lime green, or orange. These colors tend

to stimulate the appetite. Food offered on white or pastel plates is less appealing to hearty eaters.

10. Don't skip meals. You'll only overeat later.

11. Learn to distinguish appetite from hunger. When the urge to eat hits, wait several minutes to see if it passes.

12. Combat the candy habit. Instead of eating a piece of candy, brush your teeth. The tingling of the toothpaste may make your craving go away.

13. Bring your lunch to work whenever possible. You have more control when you prepare your own food instead of leaving it up to a chef.

14. Diet with a buddy. Many successful fat-loss programs rely heavily on support groups. Start your own, even with just one other person.

15. Cut back on your evening TV. Studies show that people who watch a lot of TV tend to be overfat. Heavier people agree that TV encourages them not only to sit still but to snack as well.

16. Have a carbohydrate-rich food, such as a bread slice or cracker, before bedtime to cut down on late-night cravings. Keep an orange slice or a glass of water by your bed to quiet the hunger pangs that wake you up.

17. Suck on a pickle or a lemon if you feel that you're about to binge.

18. Keep plenty of crunchy foods such as raw vegetables and air-popped popcorn on hand for emergencies. They're high in fiber, and they're filling.

19. Lose fat for yourself, not for your spouse or your friends.

20. Switch your late-night snacks to early breakfasts. Studies show that people who eat 2,000 calories in the morning lose slightly more weight than those who eat the same amount at night.

21. Skip the coffee breaks at work, especially if they mean more than coffee. Take a brisk walk instead.

22. Freeze fresh fruit such as grapes, blueberries, or strawberries. They'll take longer to eat and you'll be satisfied with less.

23. Sip hot soup. A bowl of low-calorie soup can be wonderfully filling.

24. Substitute plain yogurt for mayonnaise and sour cream in dips and dressings and on baked potatoes.

25. Avoid boredom. There is probably no bigger diet buster. Too often time on your hands translates to food in your mouth. Keep busy.

26. Know your fast food. The difference between a three-piece Kentucky Fried Chicken dinner and a McDonald's hamburger is 660 calories. Understand your calories when you pull up to any drive-in window.

27. Chew sugarless gum for oral gratification. You may find it helpful in ending a meal, too.

28. Think of meat as a condiment on vegetables, grains, or pasta, rather than the other way around. Buy smaller quantities and cut it up to add to fiber-rich main dishes.

29. Give away the "fat clothes" in your closet. Keeping larger sizes around undermines your confidence in being able to maintain your fat loss.

30. Sit straight and stand tall. Proper posture burns more calories than slouching, in addition to making your belly look smaller.

31. Turn down the volume. Your stereo could be fattening: loud noise produces stress chemicals that may make people overeat.

32. Bulk up with muscle, not fat. A pound of muscle burns 75 calories a day, a pound of fat burns only 2. Keep your muscles strong.

# _= 21 =_
# After 32 Days

One of two things will occur after 32 days. Either you'll reach your goal, in which case you'll want to maintain your fat loss and muscle gain; or you'll have additional fat to lose and need to continue.

This chapter reviews how to continue with the program to improve your results, and how to successfully make the transition to long-term maintenance.

## CONTINUING
## THE PROGRAM

If you haven't reached your goal, there is no reason you shouldn't continue with the 32/32 program for another month. The second time through, it's not necessary to begin Day 1 on the first day of the month. The experience of having gone through the program should make the second time much easier.

One suggestion, however. Take three or four days off from dieting and exercising before starting again. The rest will give your body and mind a needed diversion. Don't gorge on food. Simply eat 400 to 600 more calories per day than you were eating on the plan. Total calories should be in the range of 2,000 per day.

After three or four days, you might be surprised how anxious you are to repeat the 32-day course.

The men featured in this chapter—Zack Tannery, Jay Bobbitt, and Mark Sandberg—achieved outstanding results in back-to-back 32-day programs. Zack and Jay, in fact, did even better the second time, as every leaner day their motivation and discipline increased.

You can achieve results similar to Zack's and Jay's. Simply turn back to Chapter 13 and follow the 1,500-calorie-a-day menus for another 16 days.

Then, descend once again to 1,400 for Days 17-32, as described in Chapter 14.

I've seen several men follow the program for as many as four consecutive sessions to reach their target goals. And none of them became bored with the food choices.

It is possible to design some of your own meals to add variety to the standard menus. Just be sure your daily calories remain at the appropriate level, which necessitates a basic understanding of the four food groups, servings, and calories.

What about your exercise routine? Whether you're using Nautilus or free weights, keep your exercise routine generally the same. One set of ten exercises performed three times weekly should produce outstanding results for many months. Strive constantly to improve your muscle-to-fat ratio. You should be able to add several pounds of calorie-burning muscle to your physique each month.

Train hard and train briefly. Your progress will continue to impress you.

## MAINTAINING
## YOUR RESULTS

Once you reach your goal, your next task is to maintain your present body weight, waist size, and strength level. Doing so requires what you've now become accustomed to: sensible eating and regular exercise.

On the 32/32 maintenance plan, you must still be calorie-conscious. After completing the program, most men between 30 and 50 should be able to maintain their weight on 1,800 to 2,500 calories a day. The most practical way to determine your personal calorie needs is through trial and error. Let's begin by examining the maintenance guidelines for calories.

## MAINTENANCE GUIDELINES FOR CALORIES

| FOOD | FOR 1,800 CALORIES | FOR 1,900 CALORIES | FOR 2,000 CALORIES | FOR 2,100 CALORIES | FOR 2,200 CALORIES |
|---|---|---|---|---|---|
| **MEAT GROUP** | 3+ servings for a total of 9 ounces cooked weight | 4 servings for a total of 10 ounces cooked weight | 4 servings for a total of 10 ounces cooked weight | 4 servings for a total of 10 ounces cooked weight | 4+ servings for a total of 12 ounces cooked weight |
| **MILK GROUP** | 2 cups of whole milk 1 cup skim milk | 2 cups of whole milk 1 cup skim milk | 2 cups of whole milk 2 cups skim milk | 2 cups of whole milk 2 cups skim milk | 2 cups of whole milk 2 cups skim milk |
| **FRUITS AND VEGETABLES GROUP** | 6 servings | 6 servings | 6 servings | 6 servings | 6 servings |
| **BREADS AND CEREALS GROUP** | 6 servings | 6 servings | 6 servings | 7 servings | 7 servings |
| **OTHER FOODS** | 3 servings | 3 servings | 3 servings | 4 servings | 4 servings |

| FOR 2,300 CALORIES | FOR 2,400 CALORIES | FOR 2,500 CALORIES | NOTES |
|---|---|---|---|
| 4+ servings for a total of 12 ounces cooked weight | 4+ servings for a total of 12 ounces cooked weight | 5 servings for a total of 13 ounces cooked weight | Choose lean, well-trimmed beef, veal, lamb, and pork. Poultry and fish should have the skin removed. One egg can be subsituted for one serving of meat. One ounce of lean meat = 60 calories. |
| 2 cups of whole milk 2 cups skim milk | 2 cups of whole milk 2 cups skim milk | 2 cups of whole milk 2 cups skim milk | Two cups of milk means two 8-ounce measuring cups. One cup of skim milk = 100 calories. One cup of whole milk = 150 calories. |
| 7 servings | 7 servings | 8 servings | One fruit serving = 1 medium fruit, 2 small fruits, 1/2 banana, 1/4 cantaloupe, 10-12 grapes or cherries, 1 cup fresh berries or 1/2 cup fresh, canned, or frozen unsweetened fruit or fruit juice. Include one citrus fruit or other good source of Vitamin C daily. One fruit or vegetable serving = 50-75 calories. One vegetable serving = 1/2 cup cooked or 1 cup raw leafy vegetable. Include one dark green or deep yellow vegetable or other good source of Vitamin A at least every other day. |
| 7 servings | 8 servings | 8 servings | One serving = 1 slice of bread; 1 small dinner roll; 1/2 cup cooked cereal, noodles, macaroni, spaghetti, rice, cornmeal; 1 ounce (about 1 cup) ready-to-eat unsweetened iron-fortified cereal. One bread-cereal serving = 75 calories. |
| 4 1/2 servings | 4 1/2 servings | 4 1/2 servings | One serving = 1 teaspoon butter, margarine, or oil; 6 nuts; 2 teaspoons salad dressing or 35 calories or less of other fluid. |

Your maintenance calorie level is calculated by adding calories *gradually* to 1,500 calories a day. You might try consuming 1,800 calories a day for a week, keeping accurate records of your daily body weight. If you continue to lose and are not interested in reducing further, go up to 2,000 calories. If at 1,800 you gained slightly, adjust downward in small increments.

When your body weight remains stable for at least two weeks, you'll know the number of calories that it takes to maintain your ideal weight.

By using the maintenance chart to monitor your menus, you can keep your calories well balanced among the four food groups. This type of eating plan is one you can use comfortably for the rest of your life.

Another maintenance consideration is how you really feel about your fat loss. Try to be content with the progress you've made. Allowing yourself to feel good about your goals makes reaching them more enjoyable.

## EXERCISE MAINTENANCE

There are two primary differences between maintenance and strength-building routines. First, for maintenance you do not have to try to increase the resistance each week or so. If you can do 180 pounds on the leg extension machine for eight super-slow repetitions, then keep it on 180 pounds and do not go up to 185 pounds. You can maintain the 180-pound level much more easily than you can increase it. Second, you do not need to train three times a week. You can maintain your present level at twice a week. Some men even manage to maintain at only once a week, although I recommend training twice a week for several months before trying once a week.

In time, you might want to experiment with new exercises to concentrate on certain muscle groups or simply to alleviate boredom. This works as long as you continue to use the training guidelines presented in Chapter 7. For additional tips, you may want to review two of my previous books: *The Nautilus Book* (1988 revised edition) and *100 High-Intensity Ways to Improve Your Bodybuilding* (1989).

Any time you feel your strength decreasing, train harder and possibly more frequently than once or twice a week. Remember, metabolically active muscles are one of your body's best insurance policies against regaining fat.

*"*I have lost weight before, but never like this. I now appreciate the importance of strengthening my muscles.*"*

## JAY BOBBITT
### age 38

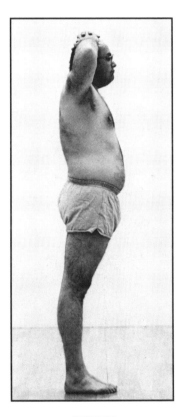

Lost
44½
pounds
of fat

Built
2
pounds
of muscle

AND
TRIMMED
8¼
inches off
his waist

in
64 days!

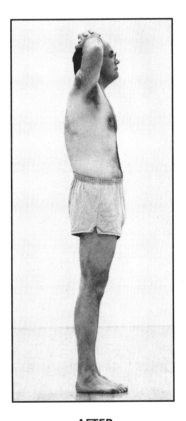

**BEFORE**
Waist Size:
44½

**AFTER**
Waist Size:
36¼

"The 32/32 course simply changed my life. I'm now a new person. Most of my aches and pains no longer bother me."

### ZACK TANNERY
**age 50**

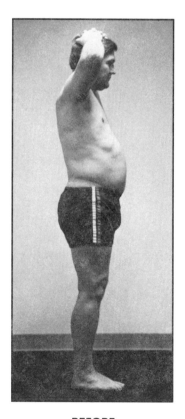

Lost
28½
pounds
of fat

Built
8
pounds
of muscle

AND
TRIMMED
4¾
inches off
his waist

in
64 days!

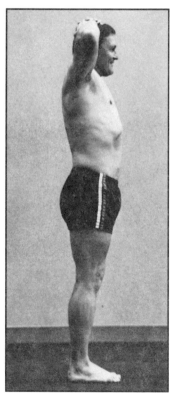

| BEFORE | AFTER |
|---|---|
| Waist Size: | Waist Size: |
| 40½ | 35¾ |

*"*I'd tried other diet programs before. Basically, I'd tried everything, so when I started Darden's program, I was skeptical. I expected to prove it was one more thing that didn't work. I was wrong. It really works. *"*

**MARK SANDBERG**
**age 36**

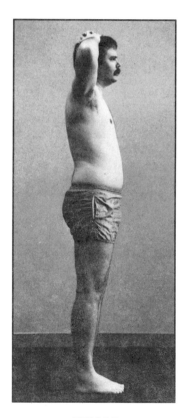

Lost
33½
pounds
of fat

Built
4¼
pounds
of muscle

AND
TRIMMED
6½
inches off
his waist

in
64 days!

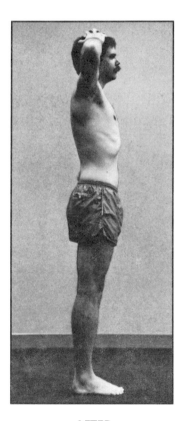

**BEFORE**
Waist Size:
38½

**AFTER**
Waist Size:
32

# _=22=_

# Questions, Comments, and Concerns

The following questions and answers should fill in any remaining gaps about the 32/32 program. Among the men participating in the plan, these concerns were fairly common.

## FUNCTION OF FAT

Q: <u>What is the function of fat in the human body?</u>

A: The primary function of fat is the long-term storage of fuel. Over 80 percent of the fuel reserve of an average adult male is stored as lipids in fatty tissue. Because of its high lipid concentration, a pound of fat contains 3,500 calories, about six times as much as an equal weight of muscle tissue. The body's fat cells provide a versatile, living inner tube, inflatable or deflatable as required, which cushions many of our internal organs. Subcutaneous fat also provides insulation.

## INCLINED TO BE FAT

Q: <u>Are some people naturally inclined to be fat?</u>

A: Genetic factors certainly play a role in a person's potential fatness and leanness. Your ability to gain or lose weight is influenced by your number of fat cells. Overfeeding results in a ballooning of these cells to several times their original size. The number of fat cells in your reserve depot seems to be determined at birth or slightly afterward and remains basically the same from that point onward. But your actual fatness or leanness is still a matter of choice—choice related to diet and exercise.

Dr. Jean Mayer, the president of Tufts University, studied the inherited tendencies of fatness while he was a professor of nutrition at Harvard University. He estimates that if both parents are obese, 80 percent of their children will be the same. If one parent is fat, the risk of obesity in offspring is 40 percent. According to Dr. Mayer, the chance of fatness is much lower, approximately 7 percent, if both parents are lean. The tendency toward fatness is probably a combination of hereditary and environmental factors.

## DOUBLE CHIN

Q: Can any special exercise eliminate a double chin?

A: There are no exercises that can eliminate the fat under your chin. Nor can exercises change how you store fat. The mechanical vibrating straps frequently present at health spas are totally ineffective. As I said earlier, spot reducing is an outright myth. The best way to combat your double chin is to reduce your overall body fat by applying the 32/32 diet and strengthening the muscles of your upper torso and neck. The Nautilus 4-way neck machine provides excellent exercise for neck strengthening.

## AEROBICS VS.
## WEIGHT TRAINING

Q: I've read that aerobic classes are much better at burning fat than weight training. Wouldn't I get better results if I added aerobics to the 32/32 program?

A: Aerobic exercise, popularly performed in class settings featuring calisthenics-type dancing set to music, is less productive than sensible weight training. While you may enjoy the camaraderie of sweating to Madonna's latest hits, beware of the following:

- There's a 75 percent chance you're damaging connective tissues in your feet, ankles, and knees. If you are performing low-impact aerobics, the damage will likely be less, but so will the cardiovascular benefits.

- Excessive aerobics may burn lean muscle tissue, especially if you're following a low-calorie diet. Doing so not only weakens you, it lowers your metabolic rate, making it harder to lose weight and keep it off.

Aerobic training is not without merit: it can improve cardiovascular condition, lower your resting heart rate, and burn extra calories. But it does none of these things significantly better than anaerobic exercise—exerting muscular force against resistance, otherwise known as weight training.

Improving your muscular strength protects your heart by reducing the levels of effort necessary to perform certain tasks. The less stressful sudden exertions are, the lower the risk to the heart.

Weight training performed with minimum rest between exercises will definitely elevate your heart rate and keep it there. Oxygenated blood will circulate throughout your body and improve your efficiency.

If the time you can devote to exercise is limited, weight training is the most logical choice. A quality aerobics program might surpass a shoddy weight-training endeavor, but if the quality of both efforts is comparable, weight training wins every time.

Too often, reputed experts assert that aerobic exercise is fueled by body fat but that weight training is contrastingly fueled by glycogen stores in the muscle. They *imply* that you can get leaner *faster* by combining dieting with aerobics than with weight training.

This is not true.

Again and again, men achieve 15- to 20-pound fat losses and 3- to 4-pound muscle gains by combining dieting and weight training for 32 days. The added muscle eventually burns more fat than a typical aerobics program.

Save the aerobics until you've significantly reduced your fat and increased your muscle size and strength. Then, if you wish to do both, do weight training and aerobics on the same day and rest the day after. You'll get much better results.

## MUSCLE NOT APPRECIATED

Q:  You believe that muscle is grossly under-appreciated, don't you?

A: I certainly do. Adult men and women have much to gain from getting as physically strong as possible, though few will ever become exceptionally muscular.

Consider that:

- Muscle functions to create movement. Your every bodily action is a result of contracting muscle. It lifts, carries, swings, runs, drives, and chews.

- Muscle adds stability and integrity to your joints, raising their level of protection against injury and subsequent pain.

- Muscle, or at least the activity of weight training, increases bone density.

- Muscle adds shape to the body. Developing your muscles is like sculpting the clay of your physique.

An article in *American Health* in November 1988 explained that "strength helps us to defy gravity and stand upright; without it, we'd be flat as pancakes frying in the sun. It's at the base of all physical skill, coordination, and balance."

There's a pound of benefit to be gained from weight training for every ounce attainable in an aerobics program.

## HOW TO BREATHE

Q: I'm confused about how to breathe when I do each exercise. What's the proper technique to use?

A: The proper breathing technique for each weight-training exercise is as follows:

- Breathe as normally as possible.

- Remind yourself to take short, shallow breaths when breathing normally becomes difficult. Do not hold your breath.

- Emphasize exhalation more than inhalation, which normally takes care of itself.

Champion powerlifters may employ unusual breathing techniques to assist their record-setting lifts, but this takes years of practice. The rest of us need to remember to keep the flow of oxygen to the muscles continual by breathing normally. The harder it is to lift the resistance, the more important it is to breathe.

Breathing makes it easier to complete those difficult last repetitions. Holding your breath does just the opposite. Many times, in fact, your breathing makes all the difference in your performance.

Holding your breath is dangerous during exercise; it can induce headache, and, should you be housing an undetected aneurysm, the consequences are all the more severe.

Breathe, breathe, breathe—during each repetition.

## ARTIFICIAL FAT SUBSTITUTES

Q: I've read several articles about low-calorie fat substitutes that may soon be available to the public. Will they be useful on the 32/32 diet?

A: Artificial fat is currently in the laboratory and under scrutiny by the Food and Drug Administration. Procter & Gamble and NutraSweet are each developing products to assist us in reducing fatty food consumption.

*Olestra*, a sucrose polyester, has been under development for more than twenty years. It cannot be digested and has no calories. Manufacturer Procter & Gamble claims that *Olestra* may soon replace conventional fats in everything from home-baked desserts to fast-food french fries and corn chips.

On the downside, however, Procter & Gamble's own tests show that *Olestra* causes tumors, liver changes, and other potentially dangerous side effects in laboratory animals. Some researchers also suspect that *Olestra* may carry fat-soluble vitamins with it through your system, causing deficiencies. It could possibly also have the same effect in the digestive tract that mineral oil has—that of a laxative.

*Simplesse* is the name for NutraSweet's "all natural fat substitute, made from either milk or egg protein." The product concept is that a gram of protein containing 4 calories can replace three grams of fat containing 27 calories. *Simplesse* can flavor ice cream, thick dips, and creamy dressings, but it cannot be used in foods that are baked or fried, as that would cause it to gel and lose its creaminess.

NutraSweet's *Simplesse* appears to be relatively safe, according to some expert impartial observers. No testing data, however, has been submitted to the Food and Drug Administration.

"If the FDA approves the new fat substitutes," reported a 1989 edition of the *Nutrition Action Newsletter*, "they could conceivably cut the risks of obesity, heart disease, high blood pressure, and possibly even cancer, by helping people eat less fat and fewer calories. Fat-free ice cream, french fries, and cream cheese could enable millions of people to reduce their fat intake with minimal effort."

On the other hand, the Tufts University *Diet and Nutrition Letter* notes: "When foods containing [artificial fat substitutes] do become available, their consumption should not be used as an excuse for bingeing on traditional fatty, high-calorie foods. They should be made part of a lifestyle that combines healthful foods with continual, moderate exercise."

As far as future 32/32 diet modifications are concerned, they await the Food and Drug Administration's ruling on the fat substitutes. This is not likely to happen until well into the 1990s, so until then, stick to the recommended menus and recipes in this book. They have been proven to produce the desired results.

## INJURY REDUCTION

Q: I seem to get injured easily in sports. Will stronger muscles help reduce my injuries?

A: Yes. Injuries in fitness activities and sports are caused by excessive force. When a force exceeds the structural integrity of the human body, an injury occurs. The logical thing for you to do is increase the structural integrity of your body. And that's exactly what proper weight training does. It strengthens your muscles, tendons, ligaments, connective tissues, and even your bones. Stronger muscles mean stronger bodies, and strong bodies withstand force much better than weak ones.

## FAT-BURNING FOODS

Q: Wouldn't your diet be more effective if it included more foods, such as grapefruit, that burn themselves up or don't turn into fat?

A: Contrary to widespread promotions, there are no such foods. Some people think that grapefruit contains enzymes which mysteriously burn up body fat. This is not true. Others believe that protein, unlike other energy sources in food, is not converted to fat. This, too, is completely false. All nutrients that provide energy contribute to the total energy pool of the food a person consumes. If the total consumed exceeds the total used, fat is formed. The body is indifferent to the sources of that energy—as a fireplace does not care whether the heat of its fire comes from pine or oak. But just as different woods supply different amounts of heat, different nutrients supply varying amounts of energy. Protein and carbohydrate each furnish four calories per gram. Fat provides nine calories per gram. Alcohol, incidentally, yields seven calories per gram.

## SWEATING AND FAT LOSS

Q: Will working up a good sweat during exercising help me lose fat?

A: Sweating does not help you reduce body fat, though it may temporarily reduce your weight. Weight loss from working up a sweat stems from depletion of water, not fat. As soon as you quench your thirst, your weight usually returns to normal.

Excessive sweating can cause your body to start preserving fat. You should particularly avoid rubber sweat suits, belts, and wraps. Even steam, sauna, and whirlpool baths can lead to problems.

Ideally you should exercise in a cool environment. A temperature between 65 and 70 degrees Fahrenheit is desirable.

## EXERCISING DURING ILLNESS

Q: What about performing the recommended exercises when I don't feel well?

A: Do not try to practice high-intensity exercise when you are ill.

Both high-intensity exercise and illness make heavy demands on your recovery ability. Illnesses can interfere with recovery from strenuous exercise, and strenuous exercise can aggravate some illnesses.

As a rule, you should rest one day for every day you are sick before resuming your weight-training program. When you start exercising again, you should lower the intensity slightly for several workouts.

## REDUCING CHOLESTEROL

Q: Will the 32/32 program reduce my cholesterol?

A: I have not performed before-and-after cholesterol testing on subjects using the exact menus and recipes in the 32/32 plan, but I have done blood work on men and women following similarly composed diets (50 percent carbohydrates, 30 percent fats, and 20 percent proteins) for six weeks. A group of 28 men I recently tested experienced the following average reductions:

- Total cholesterol     reduced 23 percent
- Triglycerides         reduced 27 percent
- TC/HDL                reduced 9 percent

In my opinion, the 32-day program would produce approximately 75 percent of the six-week results. Seventy-five percent of the above results is still a significant lowering of blood lipid levels.

## 32/32 FOR WOMEN

Q: My wife wants to go through the 32/32 program. Are there any modifications she should make?

A: Although the 32/32 plan is not designed for women, it will work reasonably well. Women differ from men in their fat-to-muscle ratios and usually have slower metabolisms. They thus require fewer calories and more time than men to achieve significant results. The daily calorie allotment of the 32/32 plan is a little high for most women seeking fat reduction. Also, the program should be extended to adapt for slower muscle growth.

A similar, but more effective, program specifically formulated for women is *The Six-Week Fat-to-Muscle Makeover*. This manual is available at most bookstores.

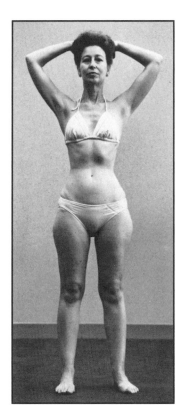 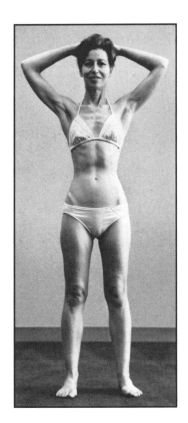

Building muscle for losing fat works for women, too. Claude Howell, age 52, went through *The Six-Week Fat-to-Muscle Makeover* twice, lost 21¼ pounds of fat, and gained 8 pounds of bodyshaping muscle. She reduced her thighs by 6⅛ inches.

## EXERCISING WITHOUT DIETING

Q: I'm satisfied with my waist size, but I'd like to put on some muscle. Can I do the 32/32 exercise routine without the diet?

A: Yes, that's exactly what I recommend you do. Adhere to the exercise routine in Chapter 18 or Chapter 19 and continue eating normally. You should be able to build from 3 to 5 pounds of muscle in 32 days, and perhaps another 2 to 4 pounds during the second month. As you get bigger and stronger, your rate of muscular growth decreases. Expect the growth rate you experienced during the first month of training to diminish slightly in subsequent months.

Two Dallas men, who were lean to begin with, had great success in building muscle. Neither practiced the diet, but both went through the supervised, super-slow, Nautilus workouts for six weeks.

Jim Shad is a 33-year-old division sales manager for Procter & Gamble. He began the program weighing 145 pounds supporting a 31¹/₈ inch waistline. Six weeks later he weighed 150 pounds, but his body-fat level had decreased from 10.8 to 8.1 percent. Jim lost 3¹/₂ pounds of fat and built 8¹/₂ pounds of muscle. In the process he lost ³/₈ of an inch off his waist and added 1³/₈ inches to his upper arms, 1 inch to his chest, and 1 inch to his thighs.

Blake Boyd's muscular waist is on the cover of this book and he demonstrates the exercises in Chapters 18 and 19. Blake was introduced to me by his father, Bill, who graduated from the 32/32 program in the summer of 1988. An aspiring actor based in California, Blake wanted to gain muscle *quickly* to balance his physique. I put him through several super-slow workouts in November 1988 before he headed back to Los Angeles to continue his training at a fitness center closer to home.

After six weeks of super-slow exercising on Nautilus equipment, Blake returned to Dallas for the Christmas holidays. I was pleasantly surprised. His body weight had increased from 171 to 180¹/₄ pounds and his body fat had decreased by ¹/₂ pound. Thus, his overall muscle gain was 9³/₄ pounds, which was evidenced by the addition of 1 inch to his upper arms, 2³/₈ inches to his chest, and 1 inch to his thighs.

Both Jim Shad and Blake Boyd demonstrated that, with proper exercise and proper diet, a man can take charge of his physique.

*"*Super-slow exercise is the best way
I know to put on muscle quickly.*"*

## BLAKE BOYD
### age 23

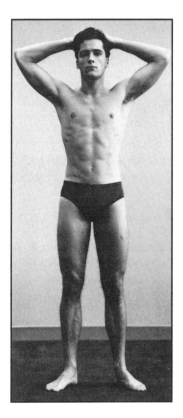

Built
9³/₄
pounds
of muscle

AND ADDED
1
inch to
his upper
arms

and
2³/₈
inches to
his chest

in 42
days!

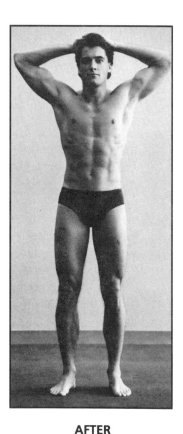

**BEFORE**
Waist Size:
29³/₄

**AFTER**
Waist Size:
30³/₄

## DIURETICS

Q: <u>Are diuretics useful in losing fat?</u>

A: The use of diuretics in the 32/32 program is strongly discouraged. Diuretics are chemicals that rid your body of excessive water. You should remember that there is very little water in fat. The weight loss from diuretics is not from fatty deposits.

 Men who self-administer diuretics may deplete their stores of potassium and other valuable substances. If too much potassium is lost, blood pressure may drop adversely, and serious problems can occur. In addition, the overuse of diuretics can irritate the kidneys or raise blood sugar.

## SKIPPING BREAKFAST

Q: <u>Is it okay to skip breakfast occasionally on the 32/32 diet?</u>

A: Please do *not* skip breakfast. Many dieters have the idea that to skip a meal means a quicker fat loss, whereas in actual fact skipping meals almost always slows down fat reduction. The reason is that when you skip breakfast, lunch, or dinner you tend to eat much more at the next meal.

## DIET SODAS

Q: <u>Is it all right to drink diet soda and eat sugarless candy and gum while on the 32/32 program?</u>

A: Some of the 32/32 dieters have used diet drinks, diet candies, and sugarless gums with great success. These treats can often satisfy a "sweet tooth" effectively. Using these products in moderation will not affect your progress.

## THOSE PROBLEM WEEKENDS

Q: <u>I find that I have no trouble dieting Monday through Thursday, but blow it on the weekends. What can I do?</u>

A: Try to convince yourself that weekends are no different than weekdays. Don't make excuses for overeating. Stick to the 32/32 diet for the required 32 days. You can certainly control yourself for four consecutive weekends. And after you've lost your excess fat and significantly increased your muscle mass, you can maintain your fat loss by eating normally once again. Recommit yourself, and hang in there!

## BREAKING THE DIET

Q: <u>I have trouble getting back on track after I've cheated. How can I handle this situation?</u>

A: Once you've cheated on the diet, the best thing is to get right back on schedule again. It's like getting back on a horse immediately after falling off. If you procrastinate you'll find it more and more difficult to get started again.

## DIETING WITHOUT EXERCISING

Q: <u>I'm not sure that my body can adapt to the intense exercise you suggest in this book. Can I do the 32/32 diet without the exercise?</u>

A: No, I wouldn't recommend it. Without proper exercise, a significant amount of your weight loss will come from your muscles. As I've stated throughout this book, building your muscles is a major factor in permanent fat loss.

   Muscle-building exercise requires the use of progressively heavier weights, or overload—and overloading your body correctly is not fun. It involves a great deal of effort on your part.

   Exercise must be demanding to be meaningful. Don't let anyone convince you that there is value in what is called effortless exercise. Effortless exercise makes about as much sense as a foodless meal!

   Decide today that you can adapt your body to both the 32/32 diet and the 32/32 exercise. Your overall results will be effective and enduring.

# —= 23 =—

# Conclusion

Not too many years ago, you could lug your pot belly to a backyard pool party and actually show it off. Mass stood for power and durability, in cars and men alike. So why not do a few cannonballs off the diving board to demonstrate your bulk?

Times have changed, and for good reasons.

Besides being unattractive, a big gut is unhealthy. It can contribute to heart disease, liver and kidney problems, diabetes, and low-back pain.

With the 32/32 program, you can flatten your belly, melt away your fat, strengthen your abdominals and other major muscles, and improve your overall health. With dedication and commitment, these things can happen quickly—in 32 days.

A 32-inch waist in 32 days is a reachable objective. Many men—just like you—have accepted the challenge, followed the instructions, and accomplished their goal.

Close your eyes and visualize your new body and your trim waist. Just think—at the next pool party you attend, you can enter the water to envious stares instead of enormous splashes.

A 32-inch waist feels great, doesn't it?

**Congratulations!**

\

# ABOUT THE AUTHOR

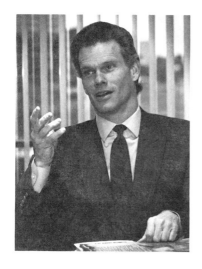

Ellington Darden's straightforward approach to exercise had its beginning during his boyhood in Conroe, Texas.

"Two minutes into my first high school football game, I broke my collarbone," Darden recalls. "That sidelined me for the season."

Not wanting to fall behind his teammates, Darden began weight training to help recover from the injury. Three years later he had transformed his six-foot frame from a lightweight 135 pounds into a 193-pound mass of muscles and energy. His progress led to a football scholarship to Baylor University and many fitness awards.

That was the beginning.

Later, Darden earned his doctor's degree in exercise science from Florida State University, where he also completed two years of post-doctoral study in food and nutrition. Today, the energetic Ph.D. is a respected innovator in exercise and nutrition, authoring more than 30 books and 300 articles on diet, weight training, and sportsmedicine.

Developing conditioning routines for men, women, teenagers, and athletes in twelve different sports, Dr. Darden's research is documented in many publications, including *The Nautilus Book, High-Intensity Bodybuilding, The Nautilus Diet,* and *The Six-Week Fat-to-Muscle Makeover.* More than three million copies of his books have been sold.

Since 1973, Dr. Darden has worked as research director for Nautilus Sports/Medicine Industries, Inc., and has conducted many seminars on the principles of strength training. These techniques have been adopted and used by fitness-minded people throughout the world.

Honored as a leader in American fitness by the President's Council on Physical Fitness and Sports in 1989, Darden's research has helped to dispel some long-accepted beliefs. "Working out for ninety minutes a day, seven days a week won't achieve any more gains than thirty minutes, three days a week," he says. "But when you tell long-time fitness buffs that they're wasting time, you can get into some pretty heated debates."

Not one to walk away from a challenge, Darden himself adheres to his format of rigorous weight training and a descending-calorie diet as a way to add muscle while reducing fat. "With additional muscle, your body burns extra calories, which allows you to return to a more normal eating plan without regaining your lost fat," he points out. "Most diets overlook that fact, and they certainly don't stress the importance of building muscle."

Dr. Darden resides in Dallas, where he continues to research and write about exercise and nutrition. "With discipline, people everywhere can improve their appearance, their strength, and their outlook on life. My goal is to make this possible for anyone willing to make a commitment."

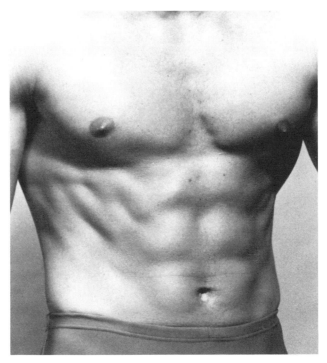

**Get a 32-inch waist in 32 days.
Do it now!**